Kidney to Share

A volume in the series

The Culture and Politics of Health Care Work
Edited by Suzanne Gordon and Sioban Nelson

For a list of books in the series, visit our website at
cornellpress.cornell.edu.

Kidney to Share

Martha Gershun
and John D. Lantos, MD

ILR Press, an imprint of
Cornell University Press

Ithaca and London

First published 2021 by Cornell University Press

Printed in the United States of America

Library of Congress Cataloging-in-Publication Data

Names: Gershun, Martha, author. | Lantos, John D., author.

Title: Kidney to share / Martha Gershun and John D. Lantos, MD.

Description: Ithaca [New York] : ILR Press, an imprint of Cornell University Press, 2021. | Series: The culture and politics of health care work | Includes bibliographical references and index.

Identifiers: LCCN 2020056163 (print) | LCCN 2020056164 (ebook) | ISBN 9781501755439 (hardcover) | ISBN 9781501755453 (pdf) | ISBN 9781501755446 (epub)

Subjects: LCSH: Gershun, Martha. | Donation of organs, tissues, etc.— Social aspects. | Donation of organs, tissues, etc.—Moral and ethical aspects. | Organ donors—United States—Biography.

Classification: LCC RD129.5 (print) | LCC RD129.5 (ebook) | DDC 362.17/83—dc23

LC record available at https://lccn.loc.gov/2020056163

LC ebook record available at https://lccn.loc.gov/2020056164

For Ann, of blessed memory,
and Cheryl, who paved the way with
courage and grace

And Don, who made the mitzvah possible
—Martha

For my daughters, Hannah, Tess, and Emma,
whose altruism and compassion inspire me
—John

Whoever saves a single life is considered to have saved the whole world.

Mishnah Sanhedrin, Talmud

Contents

Acknowledgments

There is no way to write a book about donating a kidney without acknowledging the intimate partnership such an act creates with the person receiving the organ. Deb Porter Gill is the only person on earth who, literally, has a piece of me inside her. I will always be grateful that I "matched" with this warm, smart, funny, extraordinarily strong woman. I owe a great debt to the friends and family who supported me during the kidney transplant process and helped as I struggled to shape this narrative: Jim Abel, Dr. Susan Brandt, Rob Chilson, Kay Heley, Perri Klass, Gail Lozoff, Mary McClure, Lois Rice, Linda Zappulla, and my children, Nathan Goldman and Sarah Goldman, two of the finest writers I know. And, of course, John Lantos, who agreed to help me tell the story.

—Martha

Special thanks to Children's Mercy Hospital in Kansas City, Missouri, which had the vision and the values to start a pioneering pediatric bioethics center. The leaders—Mike Artman, Fred Burry, Karen Cox, Paul Kempinski, Rand O'Donnell, Charlie Roberts, and David Westbrook, shaped an institution committed to the highest ethical principles and the best care for children. My colleagues in bioethics—Paul Bauer, Brian Carter, Jeffrey Colvin, J. C. Cowden, Jeremy Garrett, Mary Hudson, Angie Knackstedt, Laura Miller-Smith, Jennifer Pearl, Hank Puls, Dane Sommer, Vanessa Watkins, and many others—were always there for conversation, cross-covering, struggling together with tough issues, teaching, writing, and supporting each other. And to Martha, whose altruism is inspiring.

—John

Kidney to Share

Introduction

John D. Lantos, MD

This book presents two very different perspectives on living organ donation. I am a physician and bioethicist. I study, teach, and write about ethical issues that arise in medical research and practice of medicine. Martha is a Harvard MBA who left the business world to work in the not-for-profit sector. The two of us are friends, colleagues, and members of the same synagogue. In 2018, Martha decided that she would donate a kidney to a woman she read about in the newspaper.

When Martha first told me about her interest in donating a kidney to a stranger, she was excited, eager to get started; she assumed that, if she was a biologic match, then the rest would be relatively easy. She understood nothing about the long and complicated evaluation process for living donors.

I wondered whether she really understood what she might be getting into. I was intrigued to learn more about her motivation and her enthusiasm. I was concerned that she didn't understand the risks or the costs.

Martha expressed surprise at my hesitation and hastened to explain her motivation. One of her closest relatives had received a living kidney donation many years before. She and her entire family were deeply moved by the donor's generosity and deeply grateful that their loved one's life was saved. Those events shaped her conscience around the decision to donate. She was exhilarated by the prospect of continuing that story, of paying forward the generosity that had extended her cousin's life. She found the idea of giving a kidney to save someone deeply compelling. She was as puzzled by my reticence as I was by her enthusiasm.

In the months that followed, we talked often about her experience going through the process to become an organ donor. We became fascinated by the biological, legal, ethical, economic, and sociological complexities of this very strange medical procedure. I learned a lot about how the institutional structures in transplant centers work today. She learned a lot about how the history of organ donation shaped current policies and practices. Over those months, we talked about the origins of transplantation, the scientific discoveries that made it successful, the changes in the way transplant programs think about and screen living organ donors, and the ethical implications of these complex and interrelated issues.

The fact that one person's organs can be successfully transplanted into another person represents one of the most remarkable medical breakthroughs of the twentieth century. This breakthrough was a scientific triumph, but the benefits could not have been achieved with science alone. Transplantation also raised complex spiritual, legal, and ethical issues that had to be addressed. Some of these issues deal with the most profound questions facing humanity. What do we owe one another? Are there limits to altruism? If we can donate body parts, why can't we sell them? When is someone really and certifiably dead?

This book tells the story of one kidney transplant. The transplant was from a living donor. The donor was unrelated to the recipient and, when she volunteered to donate, she did not even know the recipient. This type of "altruistic donor" transplant is rare in America today. Of the nearly forty thousand transplants in the United States in 2019, only a few hundred were from unrelated living donors ("Transplants by Donor Type" n.d.).

The story we tell is important for two reasons. First, it might inspire some people to follow Martha's path and donate. The need is there. There are not enough organs to go around. More than 112,000 men, women, and children are currently on waiting lists for organ transplants in the United States. Twenty-two of them will die every day because they did not get a transplant in time ("Organ, Eye and Tissue" n.d.). The greatest need is for kidney donors. More than 80 percent of those on the transplant waiting list need a kidney ("Kidney Transplant Waiting List" n.d.). Increasing the number of organ donors, especially kidneys, will save lives—lots of lives.

This improvement in health outcomes costs us nothing; in fact, increasing the number of kidney donors, in particular, would also save money—lots of money. Kidney transplants are much less expensive than dialysis, even including the lifetime cost of immunosuppressant medications that recipients require. For a kidney patient on dialysis, the financial break-even, whether for the patient, the insurance company, or Medicare, occurs within the first two years, and the economic savings continue every year after that (Jarl et al. 2018). Unlike so many other medical interventions, increasing the number of organ transplants actually reduces the amount of health care spending required to save lives.

The second reason our story is important is that it might goad transplant programs into rethinking their processes for cultivating, evaluating, and then stewarding organ donors. These are not traditional patients even though they undergo an operation. They are not sick, though the procedure itself can cause health problems. Instead of being treated as a unique subclass of patients, they might best be treated as a unique subclass of philanthropists who are making a very, very valuable gift to the hospital, to the patient, and to society as a whole. Today, neither transplant centers nor public policy treats them that way.

Donating an organ is an act of great altruism. Donors should be encouraged and perhaps rewarded for their willingness to give a body part to save another human being. But, as this story will show, that does not always happen. For a variety of reasons including organizational complexities, bureaucratic red tape, and an extreme aversion to risk, people who want to donate face numerous barriers, hassles, and costs. If we truly want to increase the supply of organs, we need to find ways to make the process of become a living donor a lot smoother.

Martha's story occurred at an important time in the history of organ transplantation. In the early days of transplantation, the procedure was very risky. Most recipients either died or had life-long complex health problems. Today, with advances in matching and immunosuppression, most do well. As a result, transplants have become much more common and almost routine.

In 2019, in the United States, 19,267 people, living and dead, donated their organs in an effort to save the lives of others ("Organ Donation Again Sets Record in 2019" n.d.). More than 80 percent of these donated organs came from people who died. The other 19 percent—7,397 in 2019—were donated by living people.

Tragically, those numbers will likely be reduced in 2020 due to COVID-19. Transplant centers across the country canceled living donor surgeries in the earliest weeks of the pandemic in order to preserve personal protective equipment and reduce the strain on hospital capacity. In a national survey conducted the week of March 24, more than 70 percent of responding transplant centers reported complete suspension of living donor kidney transplants (Boyarsky et al. 2020). By May 4, the number of living kidney transplants performed in 2020 was 34 percent less than the comparable number in 2019. While living kidney transplants returned to near pre-pandemic levels as hospitals resumed elective surgeries, little progress had been made in recouping these significant losses five months later. As of August 22, 2020, there had been 3,167 living kidney transplants performed in the United States, compared to 4,509 on August 22, 2019, a reduction of 30 percent (for these year-to-date figures, see "Current State of Organ Donation and Transplantation" 2020).

Living donors can only give certain organs—kidneys or portions of livers, lungs, or pancreas ("Organs" n.d.). Deceased donors can provide any and all organs. One person might be able to donate two kidneys and two lungs, as well as their liver, pancreas, heart, skin, corneas, and intestines (HRSA n.d.).

Since deceased donors can often give more than one organ, this resulted in 39,717 organ transplants in 2019, the seventh consecutive annual record (HRSA n.d.). Kidney transplants are the most common. They make up 59 percent of all transplants. Livers (22 percent) are next ("More Transplants Than Ever" 2020). While each of these individual gifts is beyond measure, their aggregate impact still falls far short of the number needed for people whose organs fail every year.

The progress in transplantation could not have occurred without careful study and progress on both the biological issues and the legal and ethical issues associated with it. As an example, the concept of "brain death" was developed in the 1960s to allow organs to be taken from people whose hearts were still beating and who thus could not be declared dead by traditional cardiorespiratory criteria (Truog and Robinson 2003). Prior to the notion of brain death, people whose hearts were beating were considered to be alive, and it would have been considered murder to remove a living person's beating heart. After brain death was introduced, people could be declared dead if they had irreversible cessation of brain function, even if their hearts were still beating. This was a radical and controversial legal innovation. Some religions still do not accept the concept of brain death. A recent article in the *New Yorker* magazine summarized the controversy by quoting several prominent bioethicists. Peter Singer, a philosopher at Princeton University, described brain death as "a concept so desirable in its consequences that it is unthinkable to give up, and so shaky on its foundations that it can scarcely be supported." This new death was "an ethical choice masquerading as a medical fact." Philosopher Daniel Wikler wrote of the concept of brain death, "I thought it was demonstrably untrue. But so what?" (Aviv 2018).

Another fundamental bioethical issue in organ transplantation was the challenge of deciding whether it was ever ethically acceptable to remove an organ from a living donor. There were many good reasons to prohibit such a procedure. After all, living donation requires doctors to perform invasive and possibly risky surgery on a healthy person. Doctors must remove a fully functional organ and do it not for the benefit of the person who is undergoing that surgery but for the benefit of someone else. This would seem to violate the most fundamental principle of medical ethics: do no harm. The possibility of successful organ transplants raised a new conundrum: could the opportunity to save another person's life override this basic tenet?

This was an important question because organs from living donors offer many advantages over organs from deceased donors. They allow for greater flexibility in surgical scheduling, avoiding the last-minute rush associated with cadaveric organ transplants.

When the donor is a biological relative, living organ donations offer the potential for a better immunological match. And, in the case of kidneys, organs from living donors offer better medical outcomes for the recipient (Wang, Skeans, and Israni 2016). Most importantly, they increase the supply of available organs for everyone, since a patient who is on the waiting list for a cadaveric kidney and who then gets a kidney from a living donor comes off the waiting list. When that happens, everybody else moves up a spot, taking them closer to the top of the list to receive a transplant. Patients who would otherwise die waiting for a deceased donor will live because someone donated a living organ.

The benefits to the recipient of receiving a living organ donation are clear. But what about the donor? While the risks of organ donation are statistically very small, all living donors choose to undergo major surgery and possibly compromise their own long-term health. There may be short-term or long-term psychological consequences, as well ("Living-Donor Transplant" n.d.). In order to avoid these negative outcomes, medical centers have rigorous standards in place to ensure that only very healthy, stable people, those who are unlikely to be harmed physically or psychologically by the procedure, are approved to donate. These policies and practices seek to limit the risks of living organ donation. But they cannot erase them altogether.

In the early days of transplantation, before we understood the immunology involved and the pharmacology of immunosuppression, the only successful transplants were from close relatives. Eventually, as this book will discuss, the criteria for who could donate were expanded. With each expansion, new ethical questions arose about the motivations of donors, the prerogatives of surgeons, and the acceptable levels of physical and psychological risks for donors.

Today most living donors are relatives, life partners, or close friends of their recipients. When such relationships exist, it is easy to imagine that the donors experience psychological benefits from donating to save a loved one. That psychological benefit was important in legal and ethical debates about the acceptability of living organ donation. Doctors, judges, and ethicists argued that the physical and psychological risks of the donation were balanced by other psychological benefits to the donor.

But many people who need an organ do not know anyone who is willing to donate. Or, if they do, that person may not be healthy enough to undergo the procedure. Or that person might not be a good immunological match. In the past, those patients had to wait for a cadaveric organ. Many died before an organ became available.

In recent years, a new group of living donors have stepped up to help those with no relative or close friend to donate. Some have no prior relationship with the recipient at all. Last year, 6 percent of living organ donations came from such "altruistic donors" ("Transplants by Donor Type" n.d.). These people chose to give the gift of life to a total stranger.

The process of becoming a living donor can take months, sometimes years. It is time-consuming, invasive, and inconvenient, with dozens of players and even more moving parts. It can also be expensive. While the costs of both the evaluation and the surgery are covered by the recipient or their insurance, the costs of travel, childcare, and time off work for both the donor and their caregiver are not. These expenses can mount up. Out-of-pocket costs are likely to be especially high if the surgery is performed far from the donor's hometown, which is often the case. Not every community has a medical center equipped to perform organ transplants, and recipients must first receive approval to enter the transplant program at a center that can meet their specific medical needs. So donors must travel to the transplant center that is treating "their" recipient, both for evaluation and screening, as well as for the transplant surgery, increasing both the inconvenience and cost of donating.

In addition to increasing the burden on all living organ donors, these choices place particular hardships on people with lower incomes, who are less likely to donate organs than people with financial means (Gill et al. 2013). As a result, low-income patients are less likely to find a living donor, since they are less likely to have relatives or friends who can bear the costs of missed work, travel, and childcare (Lentine and Mandelbrot 2018).

Given the desperate need for organs, and organs from living donors in particular, one might imagine that medical centers would have policies and procedures in place to make it as easy as possible for people to be screened, and, once approved, to donate. One might imagine that public policies would encourage, protect, perhaps even reward people who offer to give the gift of life that organ donation represents. One might imagine there would be compensation for time lost from work for the evaluation and the transplant surgery and recovery for both the donor and their caregiver. One might imagine that out-of-pocket expenses, such as travel and childcare, would be reimbursed. In fact, as we shall show in this book, this is not the case at all. Both current medical center practices and public policies do very little to ameliorate the obstacles that impede healthy people who want to become living donors, even when they are deeply committed to doing so.

This problem is not unique to the United States. No health system in the world has developed an adequate systemic approach to reducing these barriers.

In recent years, the federal government has taken baby steps to ease the burdens on living donors. The federally funded National

Living Donor Assistance Center provides funds to offset some of the costs associated with donating an organ for those living in poverty. In 2019, President Trump issued an executive order that raised the levels of funding for such programs, increasing the number of donors who are potentially eligible for assistance and allowing reimbursement not just for transportation and medical expenses but also for donors' lost wages and childcare ("HSS Launches" 2019). We do not yet know what effect these changes will have, but we do know they will impact only a small percentage of potential organ donors and their recipients.

In this book, we give a detailed account of one living donor's experience. In order to understand that experience, we explore the history, the science, and the ethics of organ donation. We explore ways to ease the burden on people who are healthy and eager to donate. And we discuss the most profound question of all: How far should society go to use one person's body parts to save the life of another?

We hope that our two perspectives—one very specific and personal and one shaped by a lifetime of professional study and experience—will lead to a better understanding of the evolution and current state of organ transplantation, as well as consideration of practices and policies that could increase the willingness and ability of more people to donate.

The format of this book mirrors our conversations. Martha tells her story, and I comment on the medical and bioethical background that helps explain some of the policies, procedures, and practices that she encountered along the way.

We start with Martha's story.

1

Why Not Me?

(MARTHA)

On a beautiful Kansas City morning in April 2018, I anxiously waited to hear whether the Transplant Selection Committee at the Mayo Clinic in Rochester, Minnesota, was going to approve me as a kidney donor. The preceding three months had been an exhausting emotional roller coaster, with rewarding moments of elation followed by gut-wrenching setbacks and delays. I had willingly given my body and my mind over to intense clinical scrutiny, undergoing a litany of invasive physical and psychological tests. The transplant team at Mayo had examined my blood, my kidneys, my heart, my lungs, and my urine. They had reviewed our family finances and my personal support system. They had assessed my psychological fitness and probed my motivations for becoming an organ donor. Now, this team of doctors, nurses, and social workers would decide whether I was both healthy enough and sufficiently levelheaded to do something that many people consider to be irrational—donate one of my kidneys to a stranger.

Four months earlier, I had read an article in the *Kansas City Jewish Chronicle* about a woman who needed a kidney. The front page headline read, "Giving of Oneself: Member of the Kansas City Jewish Community in Search of a New Kidney." I did not know the woman, but her story spoke to me. The article detailed how Deb had been diagnosed with insulin dependent diabetes when she was a first-year law student in Kansas City. At the age of twenty-seven, she developed unrelated chronic kidney disease. By the time she was in her mid-thirties, Deb's kidneys were failing. She was put on the waiting list for a combined kidney-pancreas transplant. In 1999, six people, including Deb, received the "gift of life" from a forty-two-year-old woman who died in a car accident. The kidney-pancreas transplant cured Deb's diabetes and gave her a fully functioning, healthy kidney. She had a new lease on life.

Then, in 2017, Deb learned that her donated kidney was failing. It had lasted eighteen years—longer than the average deceased donor kidney, according to the American Kidney Fund. Her transplanted pancreas continued to function, but Deb needed another kidney transplant.

Deb could wait for a cadaveric kidney or try to find a living donor. The waiting time for deceased kidney donations was four to five years. Doctors told her she might not have that long. Her best chance for a successful outcome would be to find a living donor before she had to start dialysis. And that meant soon.

Deb immediately began searching for a living donor. When no family member matched, she reached out to the *Jewish Chronicle* to tell her story.

That story grabbed me. I read it several times, put the paper down, and went about my day. Later in the afternoon, I picked it up again and considered it very slowly. I could not shake the sense that it was going to be very important to me.

The reasons why Deb's story tugged at me were rooted in events that were part of my own family's story. Many years earlier, my beloved cousin Ann had desperately needed a kidney. Ann suffered from polycystic kidney disease, which the National Institutes of Health considers one of the most common genetic disorders in

America. The disease had killed her mother and one of her brothers. By the time she was in her early fifties, Ann's kidneys were failing. Her doctors started her on dialysis and put her in the queue for a kidney transplant. I did not know a lot about Ann's medical situation, but I understood that it was very, very serious.

I adored Ann. She was smart, gracious, generous, civic minded, and wickedly funny. I was desperately sad that she was so sick. I remember wondering what I could do to help. At the time, I did not know anything at all about living organ donation, but I thought I should look into becoming a donor.

As it turned out, that impulse did not go very far. Ann and I were related by virtue of her marriage to my first cousin Donald; we were family, but we were not biological relatives. So it was no surprise that I did not even pass the first bar; my blood type was not a match for Ann.

I was sorry that I could not be considered to donate to my beloved cousin. But I was also relieved I would not have to deal with the significant logistic upheaval such a donation might entail. My husband Don and I had our own busy, exhausting, all-consuming lives in Kansas City. We both had stressful jobs running high-tech startups. We were raising two school-age children. It would have been very difficult to take weeks off for a major surgical procedure far from home. We would have found a way to do it for Ann. But I knew it was probably best that we did not have to.

Then we got good news. A dear family friend, Cheryl, was a match, and she passed the medical tests to donate. On May 3, 2002, Ann received one of Cheryl's kidneys at the University of Nebraska Medical Center. There were a few postoperative complications, but Ann recovered and lived another nine years.

She lived to see both her daughters marry at joyous weddings we were delighted to attend, and she lived to see the birth of four healthy grandchildren. She was able to travel to Kansas City to celebrate with our family at my kids' Bar and Bat Mitzvot, and later, though growing weaker, she gathered the energy to make the trip for my mother's memorial service. We drove north for many Thanksgivings with my extended family at Ann and Donald's home during those years, and several times Don and I drove up to meet them for Omaha's greatest spectacle, the Berkshire Hathaway Annual Meeting.

I treasured those extra years with Ann, one of my favorite people in the whole world. And I was in awe of Cheryl for making those added years possible. When Cheryl spoke at Ann's memorial service in 2012, the full impact of her gift moved me beyond words. After Ann's death, I had a plaque installed with her name in the memorial room at our synagogue in Kansas City. Other than my parents, Ann was the only relative I felt moved to honor in this way.

And now I was reading a story about a Jewish woman in her fifties, just like Ann, who needed a kidney. Perhaps this was my chance to help another family the way Cheryl had helped mine.

Not the First Time

This was not the first time I had thought about donating something to save someone's life. Decades before, I had signed up for the National Bone Marrow Donor Registry when a colleague's granddaughter needed a transplant. The odds of finding a non-family bone marrow match are about one in a million, so I was astounded when I got a letter saying that my complete HLA tissue typing, which measures protein markers in the blood that must be compatible for a transplant to be successful, matched that of another patient in the registry. The chances that I would be asked to donate marrow were about one in ten.

When I called the donor registry to schedule the follow-up blood test that would determine whether I was a complete match for this patient, the nurse coordinator told me she was allowed to release the gender and age of my prospective match—a six-year-old little girl with aplastic anemia.

Even though there was still only a slight chance we would match, I began fantasizing about this young child whose life I might be able to save. What was she like? What were her parents like? What did it mean to them to learn there might be a match for their daughter?

A doctor friend told me that this little girl and I likely shared the same eastern European Jewish roots. Potential donors from this group are rare. Entire extended families were killed in the Holocaust, wiping out complete bloodlines. Jews of eastern European ancestry could well represent a dying patient's only hope for a match. I was thrilled at the idea that my bone marrow might save a Jew that Hitler wanted dead, that I might be able to stop the historical reach of the Holocaust with my own body, if only for this single child.

Three months after the first letter from the Bone Marrow Registry, I received a second. The tissue typing was confirmed. I was, indeed, a match. However, the letter continued, my patient was not ready for a transplant at the present time. I did not understand what that meant, so I called the registry to learn more. We had come this far. Why were we stalled now?

The nurse explained that we might be on hold for many reasons. Aplastic anemia can be a life-threatening condition, but it is not always terminal in the short run. The patient might be stable right now, and her doctors might be choosing to pursue other treatments before embarking on the dangerous bone marrow procedure. Or she might be doing worse, and they were trying to get her stronger in order to increase her odds of surviving a transplant. Or she might already be dead. We might never know.

I thought about that little girl often over the years. I wondered if I might get a call someday saying she needed my bone marrow. But I never did. Then, just a month before I read about Deb, I received an email from the National Bone Marrow Donor Registry: "On your 61st birthday, you will have completed your commitment as a member of the Be The Match Registry®." I had aged out; I was now too old to be a bone marrow donor.

That final communication was bittersweet. Twenty-four years had passed since I first had a taste of what it might mean for my body to save someone else's life. It had felt like a miracle. I had treasured that feeling of being special, of being unique, of being part of something extraordinary. And I was very sad to give it up. Reading about Deb made me wonder: Was this my chance to get it back?

Why Now?

Of course, I had heard about other people looking for organ donors. From time to time there were stories in the newspaper, or I would see posts on social media. There had even been a story in the *Jewish Chronicle* four years earlier about a member of our community seeking a kidney. Each time I read the stories I thought, "I hope someone can help." But this time my response was more visceral: Could that someone be me?

The timing was right. After a thirty-year career as a manager in both the public and private sectors, I had retired. Don had left his high-pressure job in the technology sector and was now running a local nonprofit. He was still very busy, but the pace was not as crazy as before. The last of our parents had died years before, leaving us with no remaining elder care commitments. Our children had both graduated from college and were nicely launched as independent adults. Our lives had finally become manageable. For the first time in my life, I truly had nothing more important to do. And my husband was available to help.

I asked Don to read the article in the *Jewish Chronicle*. I did not even have to say it out loud. He knew what I was asking. What would he think about my calling to see whether I was a match?

Don did not hesitate. He had loved my cousin Ann too, and he had lived with me through the ups and downs of the bone marrow saga. He understood why this particular mitzvah called to me. Don shared my belief in our obligation to help others. Most importantly, he was always supportive of my interests and aspirations, however farfetched. If I wanted to try to do this, he would support me.

The article listed a number for the Mayo Clinic Transplant Center. The next morning, heart pounding, I called to see whether I could donate my kidney to Deb.

Was This Urgent?

This all seemed very important and urgent to me. I assumed Mayo would be thrilled that someone had responded to Deb's plea so quickly, and, thanking me profusely, set me up for blood work right away. I pictured a nurse answering the phone, hearing my offer, and covering the mouthpiece to whisper excitedly to those around her, "Someone's calling for Deb—alert the lab!"

Instead, a receptionist perfunctorily answered the phone and, with very little preamble, referred me to the Mayo website to fill out a health questionnaire. She did not want to hear about the story in the *Jewish Chronicle*. She did not want to hear about my cousin Ann. I do not think she even knew who Deb was.

Moderately deflated—this was not going to be the high-intensity medical drama I had created in my mind—I logged on to the website and filled out the lengthy questionnaire. Then, with an adrenaline surge of pending altruism, I hit submit.

I immediately got an autoreply:

> Thank you very much for considering being a living kidney donor. We have received the online health history questionnaire you recently completed. The next step is for you to review information about living kidney donation. Please open a browser and paste the following addresses into your browser address bar. . . . You may not be contacted if another donor has already been identified. If you are selected, our donor coordinator will contact you within 5 business days.

I was nonplussed by the blunt tone in the email. Throughout my long management career, I had benefited greatly by following my parents' advice: be nice to everyone, communicate with everyone, thank everyone, even people who cannot help you right now; you never know when they might have exactly what you need down the road. It seemed odd that those tasked with procuring organs for transplantation would not even notify people if their generosity was not going to be required at the present time. It did not seem like good lead management to me.

Nonetheless, I filled out the online questionnaire as instructed. Five days passed with no contact from Mayo. I assumed that meant another donor had been identified. Perhaps this particular mitzvah was not mine to perform. I could move on.

Then, two weeks after I filled out the questionnaire, I got a voice message from area code 507. A woman named Lisa introduced herself as one of the nurse transplant coordinators at Mayo. She was calling to go over my questionnaire, provide information about the transplant process, and answer any questions.

I called back immediately.

Lisa told me that my reported blood type—B positive—was the same as Deb's. She said this drastically increased the odds that our organs would be compatible.

Lisa explained she would now be my primary contact throughout the transplant process. She reviewed the answers to my health questionnaire, confirming each one. Then she reviewed a long list of "next steps" I would have to take if I wanted to be an organ donor.

First, I would have to give permission for Mayo to share my lab results and medical information with the recipient's medical team for the purposes of determining my compatibility as a donor. Next, I would have to provide blood so the Mayo lab could confirm my blood type and run the tests to determine whether Deb and I were an HLA tissue type match. Transplant teams look for a match on six HLA markers when evaluating a donor-recipient pair ("Blood Tests for Transplant" n.d.). The odds of a nonrelative matching as a kidney donor are better than a bone marrow match, but they are still long—about one in one hundred thousand.

If we beat those odds and I miraculously matched for Deb, the next step would be to travel to Mayo for three days of comprehensive medical and psychological evaluations.

"Are you sure I'm not too old to donate?" I asked. "I recently learned you can't donate bone marrow past the age of sixty."

Lisa assured me that healthy people can donate kidneys through the age of seventy. Sometimes they are approved when they are even older if they are giving to a relative. While bone marrow from younger donors leads to better outcomes for transplant patients, age has a minimal effect on the success of transplanted kidneys. The surgery itself is relatively safe. She made it sound very matter-of-fact.

But there were some "areas of concern" on my questionnaire, she said. Would I be open to a phone conversation with one of their social workers?

That sounded mildly alarming. "What areas?" I asked cautiously.

Well, she explained, since I had reported that I sometimes talked to a psychologist, they needed to know more about my mental health.

"I just went to see her to figure out if it was time to retire," I protested. "And sometimes I go back when something important comes up that I want to talk about. It's not a serious mental health concern."

Lisa said she understood, but they still needed me to talk to the social worker. And then there was the pot.

"The pot?" I asked defensively.

Against my better judgment, I had disclosed on the online questionnaire that I had previously used recreational marijuana. That was not something I would normally have discussed. I knew that a lot of people thought using pot was degenerate. But Don and I had recently vacationed in Colorado, where cannabis is legal. I had smoked some pot and tried some edibles. I had only disclosed this because I did not know whether exposure to marijuana meant the surgery would be dangerous for me or rule out my kidney for Deb. Lisa informed me that my answer was not a medical disqualifier. But it was a psychological red flag.

"It is probably nothing," she said. "But we would like you to talk to our counselor."

"Okay," I agreed, even though it all seemed a little weird.

Three weeks passed. No word from Mayo. Then, finally, I got a call from Mary, a social worker on the transplant team. Mary was assigned to learn more about my mental health history and my possible drug use and report back.

I did my best to sound very clear, calm, and sober. Yes, I saw a therapist from time to time. No, I did not have a diagnosis. Yes, I would be happy to have my therapist fax my records up to Mayo.

Yes, I smoked marijuana from time to time. I also drank alcohol on occasion. Why was one more concerning than the other? Mary did not sound very concerned herself. But she explained that Mayo's transplant protocol required that anyone who reported using cannabis had to talk to an on-site substance abuse counselor before they could be approved to donate. Would I consent to do that?

I was annoyed. Certainly, I understood it made sense to screen out potential donors who had serious psychological risks. And I understood that substance abuse could be an indicator of exposure to HIV or hepatitis, conditions that might put the organ recipient at risk. But not everyone who sees a therapist has serious mental health issues. Not everyone who uses recreational pot leads a high-risk lifestyle. This felt more like blanket stigma than legitimate screening.

I worked hard to sound pleasant and not let Mary hear the annoyance in my voice. I did not want to be labeled a troublemaker or be excluded for being a jerk on the phone. In addition to faxing over my therapist's records, I agreed to talk to the substance abuse counselor.

Each of these steps seemed like one more gratuitous obstacle, delaying the transplant that might save Deb's life.

But I was starting to understand that I was one very small cog in the large bureaucracy that makes up a major transplant center. Mayo has the largest living kidney transplant program in the country ("Transplants by Donor Type, Center." n.d.). At any given time, its teams are evaluating dozens of potential living donors. I was just one of many potential donors in a long queue waiting to be processed.

My transplant might have been business as usual for Mayo, but it was certainly not for me. Like a low-level buzz, the thought of becoming a living kidney donor was a constant undertone. I was in the first year of "retirement." There were many interesting opportunities coming my way—travel, board memberships, volunteer roles. I found myself evaluating each one in light of the possibility that I might have to drop everything on a moment's notice and head to Mayo for surgery. The uncertainty and the waiting might be an inevitable part of the donation process, but I felt no one appreciated the toll they exact on potential donors.

A few days after my conversation with the nurse transplant coordinator, I was having brunch with a close friend from my synagogue. I was surprised to learn that she, too, had seen the newspaper story about Deb and that she, too, had contacted Mayo and told them that she was willing to donate. Her story took a different turn. She was not a blood type match for Deb. Mayo had notified her by email without so much as a courtesy thank-you for considering becoming an organ donor. We both agreed that the communication from Mayo did not feel like a best practice protocol.

My friend also knew a lot more about Deb than I did. She told me that Deb lived in Fort Lauderdale now, but when she lived in Kansas City she had belonged to our synagogue, and her daughters had been in the same religious and Hebrew schools that our kids had gone to years before. Her parents and siblings still lived here. In fact, Deb's father had once been on the board of our local Jewish Family Services agency, the nonprofit where my husband was now CEO, and Deb's sister-in-law knew Don from his work in the Jewish community. Our paths had likely crossed a million times though we had never met.

The whole series of events—my previous match as a bone marrow donor, my cousin Ann's kidney transplant, my recent retirement, the newspaper story about Deb, and now learning about these connections—was making it all feel oddly fated. I was very eager to move this process forward and find out for sure.

2

The Arcane Process of Screening Living Donors

(JOHN)

Martha was learning about a system for screening donors that had evolved over the decades since living donation began. She was learning that lots of people are wary about the motives of people who want to give a part of their body to a stranger. Such donations raise the deep suspicions of doctors, bioethicists, judges, and, well, ordinary people. For many years, people who wanted to donate an organ were discouraged from doing so. Today, they are tentatively welcomed, but there are remnants of the old suspicions in the extraordinarily careful medical and psychosocial screening that is required of living donors. Unfortunately, transplant programs do not usually explain this history to potential donors. As a result, donors face a series of hurdles during the evaluation process that seem arbitrary or unnecessary. Understanding history can make the screening process more comprehensible.

Doctors generally ask potential kidney donors two questions. First, they ask, do you really want to do this? That is to make sure that the donation is voluntary. Then they ask why. That is to see whether the donors can tell a story that makes sense about why they are willing to put themselves under the knife to help someone else. Clinicians instinctively doubt that anybody is truly that altruistic and see their job as figuring out what other motives, or what other psychopathology, is at work.

When the living donor is a close relative, the motives seem clear. In those situations, donors want to help a loved one because, well, because they love them. Many people are often willing to make extraordinary sacrifices to save the life of a family member. That seems "normal" and understandable.

Still, in the early days of transplantation, even donations from relatives were scrutinized carefully. Pioneers of transplantation worried about voluntariness and about the possibility of intrafamilial coercion. Such concerns were heightened if the donor was a minor. Then, doctors worried that parents might be tempted to sacrifice the well-being of one child for the benefit of another. Such fears were portrayed fictionally in Jodi Picoult's novel *My Sister's Keeper* (2004), in which parents clearly loved one of their children more than another and subjected the less loved one to a series of organ donation procedures to benefit her sister.

These risks are sufficiently fraught that doctors performing early transplants sought legal protection for doing the operation. The first such case took place in 1957, when the science and clinical art of organ transplantation was in its infancy. The case involved the nineteen-year-old identical twins Leon and Leonard Masden. At that time, twenty-one was the age of majority in their home state of Massachusetts. Leon had kidney failure; Leonard was healthy. Doctors thought transplanting one of Leonard's kidneys into Leon would save his life. Their parents wanted to proceed with the transplant. Both Leonard and Leon said that they did too. But the doctors, worried about the legal implications of violating Leonard's rights, took the case to court. They wanted a judge to approve the elective operation to harvest Leonard's kidney, an operation that would subject him to some risk and would only benefit his brother. The judge called both twins to testify in court. The parents also testified. The doctors described the operation as low risk. The court had a psychiatrist evaluate the twins and issue a report. The psychiatrist said that Leonard would benefit, psychologically, by saving his brother and would be emotionally harmed if his brother died. The judge in the case wrote,

> I am satisfied from the testimony of the psychiatrist that grave emotional impact may be visited upon Leonard if the defendants refuse to perform this operation and Leon should die, as apparently he will. . . . Such emotional disturbance could well affect the health and physical well-being of Leonard for the remainder of his life. I therefore find that this operation is necessary for the continued good health and future well-being of Leonard and that in performing the operation the defendants are conferring a benefit upon Leonard as well as upon Leon. (Spital 1989, 243)

Over the years, the formulation by this psychiatrist became the standard understanding of the motivations of family donors. If they were deemed competent, and if they were biologically or psychologically connected to the recipient, and if they expressed a desire to donate, then everybody was willing to believe that the potential psychological benefits of saving a beloved family member outweighed the potential physical harms of the surgery or the loss of a kidney. Such donations were legally permitted.

In those early days of transplantation, nobody was considering living donors who were unrelated to the recipient. That was partly for legal reasons, partly for emotional reasons, but mostly for medical reasons. Scientific knowledge about immunology was not yet very sophisticated. The only transplants that were successful were those involving living donors in which the donor and the recipient were closely related. Doctors were performing cadaveric transplants from unrelated donors, but the outcomes were not nearly as good. So nobody was willing to consider donations from unrelated living donors.

The first kidney transplant took place in 1950. This was before doctors understood the immunological processes that led a person's body to reject a transplanted organ.

Forty-nine-year-old Ruth Tucker was dying of kidney failure in Little Company of Mary Hospital in Chicago (Meszaros 2018). The surgeon Richard Lawler transplanted a cadaveric kidney into Mrs. Tucker. The kidney worked for a while. Mrs. Tucker went home after a month. Then, the kidney slowly started to fail. After ten months, Tucker's surgeons operated again to see what had happened to the kidney. They were shocked to find that it had shrunk to a size of a pea. The kidney was so small that they were almost unable to find it. They removed it (Thorwald 1971). The surgeons did not know why this had happened or what the implications would be for future transplants. Luckily, during the ten months, Mrs. Tucker's other kidney recovered some function. She survived for another five years.

Over the next few decades, researchers worked to develop better ways to treat patients who were dying of kidney failure. Some doctors thought the answer was to build a machine that could do what kidneys do—filter natural toxins out of the blood. This led to the development of dialysis. Others thought that the answer lay in replacing a failed organ with a transplanted one.

The idea of replacing organs rather than supplementing them with a mechanical device has enormous intuitive appeal—after all, if it could work, then the recipients would not need to be tethered to a machine, whether internally or externally. Instead, they could make the donor's organ part of their body. That, at least, was the dream. The realty was tough to achieve.

Since the 1950s, scientists and doctors have struggled to understand the mysterious functions of the immune system and, in particular, the process by which the body differentiates between what is "self" and what is "nonself" and rejects that which is nonself. There were two avenues of exploration in the process of coming to understand immunity, immune tolerance, immune suppression, and rejection as they related to organ transplantation. One involved investigating ways to suppress the body's immune response to foreign tissue; the other involved developing a better understanding of how to choose transplant organs that would be less likely to trigger the immune response in the first place.

The technique of using drugs to suppress the immune response is fraught with risks because insufficient immune suppression will lead to rejection of the transplanted organ. But too much immune suppression will decrease the patient's ability to fight off infection. In fact, many of the first patients to receive organ transplants died of infections because the drugs that suppressed their immune systems and allowed the transplanted organ to survive also crippled the body's mechanisms for fighting off infections. This was true for both living and cadaveric kidney, liver, and heart donations, as well as for bone marrow transplants.

In the early years of this science, when transplants were undertaken and rejection ensued, the patient's hospital course and subsequent death were often horrendous. In their book, *The Courage to Fail*, the sociologist Renée C. Fox and the historian Judith P. Swazey described one such case in gory detail. The patient is identified as Mr. K, a thirty-year-old salesman with a wife and child. He received a kidney transplant from a cadaveric donor on March 10, 1969. For the first five days, he did well. After a week, however, he began to show signs of rejection. His urine output decreased and his blood tests showed signs of impending kidney failure. The doctors increased his dose of prednisone, an immunosuppressive medication. The rejection seemed to improve, and he was discharged from the hospital on March 27, two and half weeks after the transplant. He remained stable at home for a few weeks, and the doctors again lowered his dose of prednisone. A few weeks later, however, he developed signs of diabetes and a severe skin infection. He was given both antibiotics and increased doses of prednisone. The doctors were on the horns of a dilemma. Too much immunosuppression and he could die of infection. Two little medication and he would die because his body rejected the transplanted kidney. As it turned out, he developed both infection and rejection and died at the end of May. This hospital course was typical of many early kidney transplants (Fox and Swazey 1974).

Given these dismal outcomes, it is remarkable that the pioneers of transplantation persisted. One of those pioneers, Roy Calne, a British surgeon who performed some of the earliest transplant operations in Europe in the late 1960s, described the early days as a time of "terrible disappointments and sadness but occasional elation, and a gradual understanding of the factors necessary to achieve a satisfactory operation" (Calne 2008, 1775). The determination to continue the work, Calne wrote, "required a group of loyal, dedicated and above all optimistic members who could see through the repeated unhappy outcomes that eventually most of the problems would be solved" (Calne 2008, 1775).

Meanwhile, researchers were also trying to figure out why some transplanted organs were more resistant to rejection than others. Early studies in identical twins suggested that "self" was genetically defined. Identical twins did not reject each other's organs. Organs transplanted from siblings did better than organs from more distant relatives or unrelated donors. In 1968, Thomas Starzl, an American physician, researcher, and expert on organ transplants, and colleagues reported some stark statistics about the advantages of related donors. Of forty-six kidney transplants done from related donors, only fifteen patients died in the first year; 61 percent survived for four years or more. Of the people who received kidneys from unrelated donors, two-thirds died in the first year, and most survivors were dead by four years. Only two out of eighteen recipients of kidneys from unrelated donors survived five years (Starzl et al. 1968).

The prognosis began to improve as doctors came to understand the ways that bodies recognize tissue as self or other. One primary component of this new understanding was the recognition that different proteins, or antigens, exist on the surface of cells. These have been named the histocompatibility antigens.

In 1969, Dharam Singal and colleagues reported the first evidence demonstrating that the chromosomal region coding for the major histocompatibility system, including the genes controlling HLA antigens, was involved in initiating graft rejection (Singal, Mickey, and Terasaki 1969). Before that, doctors had focused only on blood types in testing for organ compatibility. The discovery of the histocompatibility system led to much more sophisticated tests to better match donors and recipients. This led to a standard of practice by which donor and recipient had their blood tested to determine whether they shared the same HLA markers. There were six such markers, so donor and recipient could share any number from zero to six out of six. The more markers the pair shared, the better the match.

At the same time the medical science was developing, patients continued to volunteer to undergo organ transplantation. Their motivations were complex. They were dying. No other therapies were available. Perhaps they thought that they had nothing to lose. One patient who was interviewed as part of a study about informed consent said, "You really have no choice. When you're drowning even a leaky lifeboat looks good" (quoted in Myers and Kuhn 1988, 64).

In addition, some may have had altruistic motivations—a desire to help future patients by contributing to the science of organ transplantation in a way that would lead to better outcomes. Critics of the process by which patients were recruited suggest that many patients did not really understand that they were signing up for a procedure that most doctors considered highly experimental. Jay Katz, an American physician and Yale Law School professor whose career was devoted to addressing complex issues of medical ethics, for example, noted that the process of recruitment of patients as recipients of organs only took place when doctors blurred the distinction between therapy and research. This, he said, led patients to consent when they did not understand what, exactly, they were signing up for (Katz 1993).

The key breakthrough in improving outcomes for liver, kidney, and heart transplants was the fortuitous discovery of a remarkable new immunosuppressive medication, cyclosporine, in the 1970s. Cyclosporine suppressed the function of lymphocytes, the white blood cells that attack tissues that are perceived as "nonself." This suppression was first shown in rodents in 1976 and first used in human transplant recipients in the late 1970s. This drug enabled doctors to control rejection without so damaging the immune system that the patients died of infections. Starzl summarized the difference in results before and after cyclosporine: "From 1963 through 1979, 170 patients were treated with conventional immunosuppression. The chances of living for a year after liver transplantation were only about one in three. Subsequently, 244 liver recipients were provided with cyclosporine-steroid therapy between March 1980 and July 1, 1984, allowing follow-ups of 1 to more than 5 years. The chances of 1-year survival were more than doubled" (Starzl et al. 1985, 336). In Europe, Calne and colleagues reported similar remarkable improvements in kidney, pancreas, and liver transplants using cyclosporine (Calne et al. 1979).

By the mid-1980s, with the advent of better tissue typing and better immunosuppression, renal transplantation outcomes were good enough that many doctors considered it to be the standard of care for kidney failure.

These developments in immunosuppression and tissue matching improved the outcomes of transplantation from both related and unrelated donors. Because outcomes were so much better than they had been in the 1950s, doctors began to consider transplants from unrelated living donors. First, they allowed spouses to donate. When those transplants proved successful, they began to allow close friends of the patient to donate. Again, with careful screening, these transplants proved to be both safe for the donor and effective for the recipient. That would set the stage for an even more ethically controversial type of donation—donation from a total stranger.

3

Meeting "My" Recipient

(MARTHA)

The team at Mayo must have been satisfied by my agreement to send over my therapy records and to meet with their substance abuse counselor because Mary called back the same day to let me know they would be sending a lab kit to my home address.

A week later, the kit showed up on my doorstep—a square box with a cold pack, glass vials with color-coded rubber stoppers, collection instructions, and an overnight return mailing label. I was directed to find a lab to draw the blood, repack the box, and mail it back. This had to be done on a Monday, Tuesday, or Wednesday, so the samples would reliably arrive during the work week, when the shipping and receiving department was open. Mayo would reimburse me for any charges for the blood draw and presumably then bill Deb's insurance.

I called my primary care doctor's office and set up a time to have my blood drawn.

I also faxed a signed record release form to my therapist. She called soon thereafter to tell me that she thought Mayo's request for my records was inappropriate and intrusive. She saw no reason to share our confidential conversations about my career, my relationships, and my family of origin. She was not going to send them my entire file. Instead, she would write a letter summarizing our sessions and giving her professional opinion regarding my mental health status. I did not know whether that would meet the transplant team's needs, but I deferred to her professional judgement.

I shipped the blood. My therapist faxed her letter. And I waited.

Another two weeks passed with no communication.

Then, on February 20, 2018, eight weeks after my first phone call to Mayo, Lisa called again. This time she actually sounded excited: Deb and I matched on all six HLA tissue type markers! We had won the one-in-one-hundred-thousand lottery.

Time slowed down while I struggled to grasp the immensity of this new information. Lisa was congratulating me, but my mind was far away, reliving the same sense of awe and excitement I felt twenty-four years ago, when I opened the letter that revealed my bone marrow had matched with a six-year-old little girl. It had happened again—a second miracle.

Lisa's voice brought me back to reality. She was detailing what would be required of me if I chose to proceed. I would have to travel to the Mayo Clinic at my own expense for a three-day marathon schedule of medical tests, information sessions, and psychological evaluations. I would need to bring a caregiver with me, preferably the same person who would be caring for me after surgery.

There would be no cost to me for Mayo's clinical services. Deb's insurance would pay.

But it would not pay for our travel expenses or any time off work. And, of course, there was no reimbursement for the intangible costs of time, effort, and inconvenience. I was not working, so that was not an issue, but Don would have to take a week off to drive to Minnesota for the evaluation, then more time off if I passed and we progressed to the actual surgery. Lisa wanted to be sure I understood what we were getting into.

At the end of her prescribed speech, Lisa posed a question that became a mantra throughout this process: Are you sure you want to proceed? This is surgery you do not need. Your recipient has other options. You can back out at any time. We will simply report you are medically unable to donate. Do you really want to do this?

In my excitement and naïveté, it all sounded very straightforward and manageable; I told Lisa I was confident we could handle everything she described. I had already cleared the decision with my family. Don understood why I wanted to do this, and he had no objections. Our kids were agreeable as well. I was surprised at the suggestion that I would even consider changing my mind. Lisa did not know me yet. Once I commit to something, I am all in. If I could do this, I would.

I told Lisa yes. I wanted to proceed. Only months later, after we had gone through the entire process, did I realize how many potential pitfalls never even crossed my mind.

I asked Lisa when they would notify my recipient that a potential match had been found.

We don't, she said. The Health Insurance Portability and Accountability Act (HIPAA) privacy rules preclude the hospital from disclosing a potential donor's name to an unrelated recipient. How and when to tell Deb would be completely up to me. In fact, if I did not want to, I did not have to inform her at all. I could remain anonymous throughout the entire process.

The phone call from Lisa was surreal. After we hung up, I wanted concrete proof I was not making the whole thing up. I logged on to Mayo's portal, and there, clear as day, was the notification in my medical file. I was an HLA tissue match "with no adverse indications." The file showed I was now designated as "#1 Potential Kidney Donor."

Though I did not have to tell Deb or anyone else, keeping this a secret did not seem like a feasible option. The Kansas City Jewish community is relatively small. Lots of people knew Deb was looking for a kidney donor. We would soon be going to Mayo for a week of testing. I did not want to lie about where we were going, and I did not want anyone to think I was seriously ill. I wanted to tell them the truth: I was going to Mayo to be evaluated to donate a kidney. It would not take long for our community to put the two stories together.

I also needed to understand the time frame we were talking about for a potential surgery date. Our son was getting married in early June. Don and I were planning to leave on an overseas vacation a few weeks after that. We had reached the point where we were about to purchase nonrefundable airline tickets. How sick was Deb? How soon did she need a transplant? Could I safely commit to our summer vacation plans? Did I need to wait?

Mayo was prohibited by HIPAA from answering any of my questions. I would have to ask Deb directly if I wanted answers.

I also felt a very strong pull to know the woman I was doing this for. I had signed up to donate to a stranger, but now that we had matched, I was keenly curious about the woman who might someday carry a part of my body.

While some living organ donors are completely anonymous—they offer to donate to the general pool and never know who receives their kidney—I fell into a slightly different category. I was still considered a stranger donor; I did not know Deb before I offered to donate. But I had read her story, and my offer was specific and directed. It was personal.

If it was possible, if it was okay with her, I wanted to meet Deb.

That turned out to be harder than I expected. We might be an HLA tissue type match, compatible on a fundamental biological level, but that did not make it any easier to find Deb's contact information. Mayo would not tell me. Her last name was very common, so an online search proved futile. I did not know her Kansas City family, and I did not think it would be appropriate to contact them before I talked to her. So I turned to that ubiquitous tool, social media. I looked her up on Facebook and sent her a message:

> Hi, Debra. Not sure if you get messages this way, but I thought I'd try. Is there an email address to contact you directly? I called Mayo after I read about your need for a kidney in the Chronicle. After blood tests, they called today to say I am a possible match—B Positive and an HLA tissue type match. They are working now to set up the 3 days of medical testing to assess my overall health and the viability of my kidney for donation. Everything seems to move slowly there—we are looking at appointments in mid-May!! Which seems like a long time to me. They said I could write to you, though they apparently don't give you any information about me. That just seemed weird, so I thought I'd reach out. Write back if you want— okay if not. I just retired as Exec Director of Jackson County CASA, so Family Law is my world, too.

It was very strange to send that message. I was initiating a different sort of relationship than I had ever had with anyone in my life. I had fantasized about the six-year-old girl who was my bone marrow match. But we never met in person. I never even knew her name. What if I did not like Deb? What if she did not like me? Would she think I was some weirdo who was stalking her? Would she be grasping and desperate, someone whose emotional needs were more than I could handle? What was I getting into? I began to think of all the ways this could go wrong.

I need not have worried. I heard back by email the next day:

> Dear Martha,
> I read your message and it literally took my breath away. I had to take a little time before responding because I couldn't find the words to express my gratitude. (And if you ask anyone, it is very

rare for me to be speechless. :-)) Your incredible offer to donate one of your kidneys to me, or to anyone you don't know, is beyond generous. It's mind boggling.

I spoke to my transplant coordinator at Mayo today and I'd be happy to communicate with you if you are comfortable with that.

You can text, call or email.

Besides the fact that we might share an organ someday, it sounds like we have a lot in common.

I hope that your week is going well and that you are staying safe and warm. I fly into Kansas City from Fort Lauderdale today and hope to get there before the next storm moves through.

Looking forward to hearing from you soon!

Deb

She was real and sounded normal, funny, practical, and nice. I was very relieved.

The next day Don ran into Deb's sister-in-law at the Jewish Community Center. Deb must have told her family about me, and they must have made the connection to Don, because Carol threw her arms around him and thanked him profusely. When Don came home from work that night and reported the encounter, I got goose bumps. Deb was real. Her family was real. The possibility of an organ transplant was real. This was no longer an idea, an aspiration, a fantasy. This was no longer a Hail Mary, motivated by my desire to honor my cousin's memory and my desire to redeem my now aging bone marrow. This was happening.

By fortunate coincidence, Deb was en route to spend a week in Kansas City when she read my Facebook message. We both agreed we should take advantage of this chance to meet in person. This might well be one of the most important meetings in either of our lives. But we tried to act as if nothing out of the ordinary was at stake. As matter-of-factly as if we were setting up a business meeting or a girlfriend get-together, we arranged a time and place for lunch.

I dressed as carefully as I would for a first date—nice, but casual, nothing too showy. I wanted to look young, thin, and healthy. Since the first two ships had already sailed, I settled for healthy.

The minute Deb walked into the restaurant, with her warm energy and big, open smile, it felt like we had known each other for years. Our lunch conversation swirled around areas of common interest: writing and publishing (aspirational), politics (liberal), sex (even more liberal), child welfare (appalled), and everyone we knew in common (a lot!). We discovered that Deb had worked as a lawyer in the Jackson County, Missouri, prosecutor's office in the child sex crimes unit, while decades later I had worked to help child abuse victims in the same jurisdiction. We discovered my long-term primary care physician had once been Deb's doctor too. As we uncovered each new bit of synchronicity, we told each other that our match was *b'sheret*, the Hebrew word for something or someone that was "meant to be."

Our conversation was practical too. Deb knew a great deal about the organ transplant world from her first experience nearly twenty years before. Her evaluation with Mayo for this second transplant had taken place months before I entered the picture, so she understood a lot more about how things worked. Over lunch, she told me how rare our blood type is—less than 9 percent of the US population is B positive—and we marveled that we had matched.

I warmed to Deb right away. I loved that she was not maudlin about her health or mawkish about my willingness to donate an organ. I loved that she was visibly grateful for my offer, but also completely appropriate, with sensible boundaries that made me feel safe. I loved that she was smart and practical and matter-of-fact. I loved that despite decades of difficult health issues, she was fun and optimistic and had a wicked sense of humor. In many ways, she reminded me of my cousin Ann.

It was also reassuring to hear Deb talk about her first organ transplant and her fierce determination to take care of her health and manage the complicated medication regimen required of all transplant recipients. Before Deb and I met, I had not thought about how I would feel if I donated a kidney to someone who was willfully reckless with their health or careless with medications. Now I could see that indications of such behavior would have made me nervous about donating. I wanted "my" recipient to take good care of "my" kidney.

I have wondered a great deal about how much it mattered that Deb was a lot like me—a white, upper-middle-class, well-educated Jewish mother of two. I would like to think that I would have been just as willing to donate to a single, childless African American man, or someone who never finished high school. Or a Muslim immigrant. Or a devout evangelical Christian.

I have also wondered how I would have felt if I had not liked Deb, or—worse—if we had held wildly divergent worldviews. I knew I did not have to feel like we could be best friends. That would clearly be too high a bar. But what if she had been a racist? An anti-Semite? A homophobe? What if she thought I was going to hell, because I was a Jew? What if she held ideas I violently disagreed with and voted in direct violation of my most cherished values? Would I have given her a kidney then?

I don't know. I never had to test the limits of my altruism in those ways. I only know that I matched to give a kidney to Deb, that I liked her very much, and that I desperately hoped I would be able to save her life.

4

Do I Own My Organs?

(JOHN)

Martha was happy and fortunate that she liked Deb. It made her feel good about donating her kidney. But what if they had met and Martha had not liked her? Would she have withdrawn the offer to donate? She certainly could have. As her narrative makes abundantly clear, and as the design of all transplant programs ensures, living donors can back out at any time and for any reason. One of those reasons could have been that Martha did not want to help this particular recipient. That could have been for any reason, including political values, lifestyle, religion, or skin color. Living donors are treated by the law and by doctors as the owners of their bodies, and their body parts are considered goods that they can donate or not to whomever they want.

That is not the way society treats organs from cadaveric donors. When an organ is procured from a deceased donor, neither the donor (through an advance directive) nor the family usually gets to dictate in advance who should receive the organs—or who should not. While family members of deceased donors are legally permitted to specify where their relative's organs should go, they are discouraged from doing so (Cronin and Price 2008). Instead, organs from cadavers are generally put into national pools and allocated according to nationally agreed-upon criteria.

Cadaveric organs are treated not as private property but as a public good. Their use is governed not by the autonomy-based preferences of the donor or the donor's family but, instead, by considerations of justice that are built into the administrative rules that dictate how organs should be allocated. And those rules are fundamentally utilitarian. The organs should go where they will do the most good. One review of the allocation rules for kidneys summarized the goal as "pairing kidneys expected to function the longest with recipients expected to live the longest" (Formica 2017).

This justice-based approach to organ allocation attempts to harmonize a number of potentially conflicting considerations. In the United States, we start from the premise that the family has the right to decide whether organs are donated or not. In that sense, family members own the body of their deceased loved one. Some countries view this differently—instead of seeking a family's consent for donation, they presume that it is permissible to harvest organs unless the family speaks up and opts out (Saunders 2012). Studies show that, with such policies, deceased donation rates rise (Ahmad et al. 2019). But such policies generate political and emotional opposition. One response to such programs, elicited in a qualitative study done in the United Kingdom, reflected one point of view: "If I donate my organs, it's a gift. If you take them, it's theft" (Miller, Currie, and O'Carroll 2019).

There are practical reasons for treating cadaveric organs differently than organs from a living donor. We cannot predict the time of our deaths. It is extremely unlikely that a loved one—or anyone we know—will need a kidney at the time we die. So, if we choose to donate, the organs will almost always go to a stranger.

There is tension between the idea that organs are the property of individuals or their families and the idea that organs are a communal good. In an article in the *American Journal of Bioethics*, Jamie

Lindemann Nelson, a professor of philosophy at Michigan State University, writes,

> We don't seem to know just what to make of organs for transplant. As things stand, organs aren't fully property as they cannot be sold, nor are they fully public goods, as society may not use them at will. The problems about soliciting directed donation correspond to this ambiguity. Suppose my organs belong to me or to my estate. We would need an argument to block my providing them as gifts to whomever I chose. Suppose on the other hand that, at my death, my organs became public goods. Then the appropriate way to distribute them would seem to be via a system of impartial, impersonal justice. (Nelson 2005, 27)

Hagi Boas, an Israeli sociologist and anthropologist who heads the Science, Technology, and Civilization Cluster at the Van Leer Jerusalem Institute, characterizes most countries' current approach to organ sharing from deceased donors as a form of "bodily communism," from each according to his good will (and his physiological state), to each according to his needs with the involvement of the state as redistributive agency (Boas 2011, 1380).

These issues are highlighted by Martha's implicit questions about her own motivations for donating. Like most living donors, she had responded to a very specific plea for an organ. She had responded to a plea from someone in her community who reminded her of her beloved cousin Ann. And the more she got to know that person, the more determined she became to go through with the transplant. She had not reached out to a transplant clinic to give her kidney to anyone who needed one. Her altruism had limits.

5

Evaluation at Mayo

(MARTHA)

Now that I had been identified as Deb's match, the next step was to find a week to travel to Mayo for the three days of required tests and evaluations. Of all the hoops I had to jump through to become an organ donor, nailing down that time frame was one of the most frustrating and stressful.

I started with the dates that would work for us. From the beginning, I had promised our family that I would not let this project interfere with our son's wedding in early June. I wanted to schedule the tests well before that joyous event. Don had several important work commitments in April, so that month was out.

Deb also had preferences. She wanted to know as soon as possible whether I was going to be approved to donate. That was particularly important because her health insurance would pay to screen only one potential donor at a time. Now that I had been designated the #1 Potential Kidney Donor, they would not even run blood tests to identify other potential matches unless I backed out or was disqualified. If I was not approved to donate, then Deb would have to start the search all over again. No one knew how long it might take to find another donor, so Deb needed me to get evaluated as soon as possible.

It was already the first week in March. Don and I had been talk-ing about going to Minneapolis to celebrate the first night of Pass-over with our son and his fiancée at the end of the month. If we could schedule the trip to Rochester for the last week of March, we could combine the two trips. It was the perfect answer.

Then Mayo said no.

They could make the schedule work, with one exception: they did not have an open slot with the substance abuse counselor. While they had available appointments during our desired week with every other specialist and clinic, Mayo's substance abuse counselors were entirely booked up for the month of March.

Could we come in April instead? No, Don had work commit-ments. Then the next available window would be mid-May, the scheduler reported matter-of-factly. No, I said. That will not work. It is just two weeks before our son's wedding; I am not available.

I pleaded with her to book us for a March evaluation. She was immovable. There were no open appointments with substance abuse counselors in March; there was nothing she could do.

The thought of traveling to Rochester for a week of testing in mid-May made me desperately unhappy. When I first talked to Mayo about donating, before I even consented to a blood test to see whether I was a match, I had told them the weeks surround-ing our son's wedding were sacrosanct. Lisa had assured me that would not be a problem, they were flexible about scheduling, and the donor's needs always took priority. That was clearly not true. The only dates Mayo would give me were threatening to distract me during the very time I wanted to focus on our family and our joy at this marriage. We had a deal, and they were already violating it.

Deb was not happy either. The May evaluation dates on offer put her in limbo for two more months. If my tests uncovered some reason that I could not donate, that delay could prove costly to her health. That one substance abuse appointment was threatening to derail our entire schedule, all because I had naïvely confessed to smoking a few joints. If I had known what a ruckus a little weed was going to cause, I would have lied.

I called Mayo again to try to negotiate an earlier date. The staff was not sympathetic. They calmly explained that a lot of departments make referrals to their limited supply of substance abuse counselors; potential organ donors receive no special consideration in vying for a spot on that calendar. I suggested alternatives: What if I saw a substance abuse counselor in Kansas City and faxed over the session notes? What if I talked with one of their substance abuse counselors via Skype? What if they tested the blood they had already collected or the pee they could collect in March to confirm that I had no recent exposure to marijuana—or to any other recreational drugs, for that matter? What if they just believed me—that this was not an issue? No, no, and hell no. It appeared nothing would satisfy the transplant team except an in-person interview with one of their own nearly-impossible-to-schedule substance abuse counselors. From my point of view, Mayo was stubbornly refusing to think creatively about a way to solve this problem, a problem they had manufactured in the first place.

I really could not see a way to get Deb a quick answer about my suitability as her donor, and I could not see a way to honor my promise not to interfere with my family's wedding plans. I was happy to volunteer to donate a kidney, but I had not signed up for this level of emotional distress. I really did not know what to do.

Then Deb came up with a solution! What if Don and I went to Mayo in March and took care of all the tests except the elusive substance abuse evaluation? Then, if there were medical barriers to my donating, we would know very soon, and Deb's team could move on to look for another donor. And if I passed all the medical tests, we would assume I was good to go. We all knew the marijuana use was not a "real" problem. We just had to check that box for Mayo. Unlike the other evaluation appointments, this one did not require me to have a caregiver. I could fly back to Rochester alone in April to take care of the one-hour substance abuse appointment. It would be inconvenient and expensive, but it was doable.

Mayo had no objection to our plan. As long as I presented myself for the substance abuse evaluation, they did not really care how much time or money it cost. They scheduled all my evaluations minus one for the last week of March and put me on the calendar for a substance abuse consult in mid-April.

Preparing for Mayo

Don and I had always assumed we would pay for the various trips involved in this process. We could afford it, and we assumed this would be part of our donation. But Deb insisted that she would pick up the tab for all our out-of-pocket expenses—for the first evaluation trip to Rochester, and a second one to see the substance abuse counselor, as well as the surgery trip if we got that far. We accepted her offer.

Naturally optimistic, I had given very little thought to the possibility that the upcoming tests would uncover some unknown condition that would disqualify me as a donor. For several years I had been getting a comprehensive annual physical from my primary care internist, complete with lab work that I was sure would have revealed any underlying health concerns. I was up to date on my PAP smears, mammograms, and colonoscopies. And since I had left my high-stress job the year before, I was working out more and felt better than I had in a long time. I figured that meant I was healthy.

I learned later that many people seeking to donate discovered during the evaluation process that there were medical reasons they could not donate. Some even had structural abnormalities in one or both kidneys. These congenital conditions were asymptomatic and would likely never create problems for the prospective donor, especially if only one kidney was affected. But it did mean donating might be too risky for them or for their recipient and they would be rejected as a donor. If I had known those details, I might have worried. But I did not know enough to obsess about that possibility. Instead I obsessed about my weight.

This was a familiar neurosis. I had obsessed about my weight my entire life. I had struggled with food, body image, and obesity for as long as I could remember, sometimes winning the fight and sometimes losing. Most dramatically, I had gained eighty pounds during my second pregnancy, battling nausea that could only be tamed with constant carbs, and developing insulin-dependent gestational diabetes. The diabetes resolved immediately after our daughter was born, but I could not seem to shed the weight. For the next twelve years I tried every eating plan, diet pill, or exercise regimen that flitted across my radar. I finally stumbled on a diet and exercise plan that worked. I lost ninety pounds and took up walking, then running. Eventually I trained to run the Chicago Marathon—twice—as well as a number of half marathons in Kansas City.

Now, a decade later, the pounds had started to creep back. I had gone up a clothing size or two and was starting to feel anxious about my weight again. I had been working out religiously since my retirement, and had been dieting aggressively in anticipation of Nathan's wedding. I was doing better again. But I still was not back to marathon form.

Starting in grade school my only defense against the nagging of parents, doctors, coaches, and friends to lose weight was a dismissive protest: "I'm happy; I'm not hurting anyone else." Now, it seemed, that might no longer be true. If my lifelong struggle with weight— my darkest, most personal humiliation—kept me from saving Deb's life, the shame would be crushing. And it would not just be private shame. After an entire adolescence and adulthood spent camouflaging my true identity with good clothes, good sex, and good conversation, I would be exposed for what I really was—a fat girl.

Alternatively, if I passed Mayo's rigorous evaluation, it would be the ultimate response to every misguided relative, snarky colleague, unkind boyfriend, and self-loathing inner voice that had felt entitled to comment on my weight. If I could do this, then my body was, indeed, worthy.

Was This Safe?

Now that things were moving forward, it occurred to me I should probably notify my primary care provider of my donation plans. I called his office and let the nurse know. A few days later, my doctor uncharacteristically called me at home, after hours. I thought he might be calling to dissuade me. I was too old. I was too fat. This was too dangerous. But, instead, he was calling to tell me he thought my offer to donate a kidney was amazing and generous and exciting. When I told him Deb was my potential recipient, he was surprised. He had been her doctor years before when she had lived in Kansas City, and he remembered her first transplant. He congratulated me on my willingness to help. He also reminded me that he had trained as a nephrologist before going into primary care and served as board chair of the local chapter of the National Kidney Foundation.

Since I had an expert on the line, I took the opportunity to address my fears. I was unwilling to ask directly about my weight, so I asked a more general proxy question instead: "You've taken care of me for over thirty years and know my health status better than anyone—do you think I'm healthy enough to do this?" Absolutely, he replied without hesitation. You are fine.

He followed up by sending me a recent paper that reviewed fifty-two other studies on the health outcomes for 118,000 adult living kidney donors over twenty-four years. I was thrilled to read there were that many people who had done this. It made the whole project feel less extreme. The living kidney donors in the study had no increased risk for chronic diseases such as type 2 diabetes, hypertension, or cardiovascular disease; no adverse psychological outcomes; and they lived just as long as everyone else. There was a slightly increased risk of end stage renal disease, although the absolute risk remained very low (O'Keefe et al. 2018).

There were caveats to those study results. As I was finding out firsthand, living kidney donors were carefully screened. People with preexisting health problems would not be allowed to donate. So, of course, those who were approved tended to have good long-term health prospects. Still, I was glad to read that kidney donors went on to live long, full, healthy lives.

The Qualifying Exams

A few weeks before our scheduled trip to Rochester, my Mayo portal started to populate with the testing schedule: fasting blood draw, twenty-four-hour urine collection, eighteen-hour blood pressure monitor, abdominal CT scan, chest X-ray, EKG, kidney function test. There were other appointments too: nephrologist, donor education class, hypertension clinic, financial counselor, surgeon, nurse transplant coordinator, social worker, dietician, donor advocate.

The tests and consultations had two purposes. First and foremost, they were designed to ensure that donating an organ would not adversely impact my medical or emotional health in either the short or long term. They wanted to be sure that I would survive the surgery and could live a full and healthy life with only one kidney. Second, they wanted to be sure that my kidney would not hurt Deb. Was it strong and healthy? Did it function properly? Was it free of tumors, cysts, and cancers? Did I carry any transmissible diseases?

The Mayo schedule came with pages and pages of instructions. Nothing to eat twelve hours before the blood tests. Limit whole milk, cream, oil, gravy, fatty meats, or fried foods. No vitamins or iron. Take your other prescribed medications. No exercise or unusual physical activity while wearing the eighteen-hour blood pressure monitor. No driving or riding in a car for more than thirty minutes. No showers, baths, hot tubs, or swimming. No sedation. No food for four hours before the renal function test. Drink two to three eight-ounce glasses of water one hour before the test, then don't pee, so that you can empty your bladder immediately when the appointment starts. Restrict your diet the night before the abdominal CT scan. No jewelry for the chest X-ray. No nylons for the EKG. No perfume for any appointments in the transplant clinic. Refrigerate your urine. Whew!

It appeared becoming a donor was going to require some pretty significant project management skills. I made a schedule in an Excel spreadsheet, color coded for eating, drinking, fasting, peeing, and driving. The completed chart was complicated and colorful. Some of the appointment connections looked pretty tight, spread over a bunch of floors in a bunch of different buildings, and my opportunities to eat and drink would have to be squeezed in between appointments and the various fasting restrictions. This would only work if we did not get lost, the providers were on time, and the lines in the cafeteria were not too long. I had a lifelong fear of being late; now I added adhering to the schedule to my list of things to worry about.

The week before our departure, another box arrived from Mayo. This one contained the world's largest orange plastic jug, labeled with a bar code, a physician's name, and my Mayo ID number; a wide-mouth plastic cup with pouring spout; and a folded piece of paper with "24-Hour Urine Collection Instructions." Starting twenty-four hours before my Mayo appointments, I was to collect every drop of my pee in the jug, refrigerate it, and bring it to the Mayo lab early the first morning of my testing schedule. We were driving to Rochester from Kansas City the day before the tests, so I would be carrying that jug into QuikTrip and Love's restrooms throughout Missouri, Nebraska, Iowa, and Minnesota. Whoever designed this process had a real sense of humor, I thought sardonically.

I asked Lisa if it would be easier if we just flew to Rochester. She reminded me of the obvious—there was no way I would get through security with that jug, clearly carrying more than three ounces of liquid. Try explaining that to the TSA agents!

The four-hundred-mile drive from Kansas City to Rochester took longer than expected, since just thinking about the urine collection process made me need to stop more often than usual. By the time we reached the Rochester Hilton Garden Inn in the late afternoon, my jug was nearly half full. We settled into the hotel to relax before the tests began the next day.

Meeting Mayo for the First Time

The day started with a pitch-dark ride to Mayo in a cold drizzling rain. My first job was to report at 6:30 a.m. to the lab on the ground floor of Charlton, one of many buildings in the huge cluster of high rises that make up the Methodist Campus of the Mayo Clinic. They would draw blood, and I would be relieved of my orange jug. There were more than one hundred other people also assigned to the 6:30 a.m. slot at the Charlton lobby-level lab. I dutifully lined up in the winding queue, reminiscent of family trips to Disney World. Eyeing the growing crowd filling the waiting room, I started to become anxious that I would miss my first "appointment." I had not yet learned what an assigned appointment time at Mayo really means. It is not an actual appointment time; it is a suggestion about when to report to a waiting room so that Mayo can manage their tremendous workflow with some semblance of order.

And there was plenty of order on display in the Charlton lab. A rotating team of dozens of phlebotomists in matching maroon scrubs cycled in from the back room with impressive regularity, calling name after name. The waiting room started to thin out. Within fifteen minutes I was ten vials of blood lighter and in possession of another plastic cup for a real-time urine sample.

For the next three days, Don and I scrambled between medical buildings—Charlton, Gonda, Hilton, Guggenheim, Mayo—all connected underground through the famed Mayo "subway" and many connected by skywalks on higher floors. We were astounded at the size and scope of the campus, really a self-enclosed city. In addition to the medical clinics and labs (we counted three), the vast complex contains retail stores (carrying gifts, flowers, wigs for chemo patients, and three pharmacies), coffee shops, fast food restaurants, amazing visual art (including a grand overhead Dale

Chihuly installation), a public performing space, and at least one grand piano. Every time we stopped to get our bearings, someone on the Mayo staff would come up to ask whether they could help. Once again I was reminded of Disney World. I suspected frequent customer service training and wondered why their customer service was so good on-site and yet could not extend to getting me a substance abuse appointment at a convenient time.

Some of the tests I had to undergo were pretty weird. For the all-important kidney function test, I had to pee every hour in a fake "commode" in the middle of an exam room in between getting injections of a radioactive contrast material, drinking bottles of water (they offered soda alternatives), having a sonogram of my bladder, and getting my blood drawn. Fortunately, other than the needle pricks for the contrast material and the blood draws, the test did not hurt.

None of the tests really hurt. Fatigue, not pain, became the issue. I started off sleep deprived from our first night in Rochester, when I kept waking up worrying about capturing my urine in the orange jug. By the second night, I was wearing an eighteen-hour blood pressure cuff, which woke me every forty minutes with its annoying buzzing and puffing. Add to that the unrelenting pace of back-to-back appointments and it was no wonder I was dragging.

Through my exhaustion-induced haze, I was nonetheless able to appreciate the extraordinary efficiency and cohesive systems that make Mayo so justifiably famous. Every exam room and testing station was carefully designed to ensure privacy, comfort, and rapid patient flow. Dozens of patients were processed in the half-hour time slot I was assigned to get a chest X-ray and even more at the clinic that handled the EKGs.

The electronic medical records system was impressive too. By the time I met Dr. Bentall, the nephrologist who would manage my case, just three hours after my first early-morning appointment at the lab, all my blood and urine tests had been run and the results posted to the Mayo portal for his review.

Handsome and Charming Mayo Doctors

Dr. Bentall was the quintessential Mayo doctor—good looking, with sparkling eyes, an easy smile, and a delightful British accent. Deb had told me on one of our phone calls that "they are all from somewhere exotic, and they are all smart and handsome and charming." She had nailed it. I liked him immediately.

Dr. Bentall's job was to ensure that I was healthy enough to donate. That included psychological health.

Dr. Bentall's first question was about my motivation to be a kidney donor. I told him about Ann and about my near miss as a bone marrow donor. I also explained I was recently retired from my job running a nonprofit that helped abused and neglected children and this seemed like a worthy way to stay useful. I was not sure what sorts of reasons would satisfy him or whether people got rejected for bad motivations.

6

Are "Stranger Donors" Irrational?

(JOHN)

Once donations were allowed from unrelated donors, questions naturally arose about the degree of emotional relationship that was essential to justify the claim that donation provided a psychological benefit to the donor. If a spouse or close friend could donate, why not a coworker, a neighbor, or a member of somebody's church? Why not the friend of a friend? Eventually, the question arose whether a total stranger could donate. In such cases, the psychological benefit, if there was one, accrued not because the donor was saving a loved one but because the donor, presumably, felt good about saving anyone they could.

Doctors and policy makers were puzzled about how to understand the motivations of people who offered to donate a kidney to a stranger. These donors' motives were so suspect that some countries outlawed such donations altogether. The United Kingdom had a law called the Unrelated Live Transplant Registry Authority. It required organ donors to provide proof that they had a relationship with the recipient. The law was a little vague about how, exactly, a relationship could be proved, or how close the relationship had to be. Potential donors would bring photographs showing them together with the recipient. Sometimes that would be enough; sometimes more concrete proof was required. The law said, in essence, that no sane person would donate to a stranger and thus that anyone who wanted to do so was insane and needed to be protected from their own absurd altruism.

Eventually, the UK law was challenged. In 2007, as recounted on the Give a Kidney charity's website, a woman named Kay Mason, a retired palliative care nurse, decided that she wanted to donate one of her kidneys to anybody who needed it. She was angry that the law treated potential donors as if they were insane. She wrote, "The thinking was that you had to be mad to want to give a kidney to a stranger. And if you were mad, you couldn't be allowed to give. But I was perfectly sane" ("Ten Years" 2017). She prevailed. The law was struck down and, in its place, the Human Tissue Act went into effect, allowing donation of organs by strangers.

In the United States, there is no federal legislation or public policy regulating stranger donors. Decisions about whether to permit these donations have historically been left to individual medical centers. Many transplant centers were initially very skeptical about accepting stranger donors. They shared the widespread belief that such people must be irrational masochists or pathological altruists. Over the years, however, attitudes began to shift, motivated, in part, by the increasing success of kidney transplants between unrelated people. Further motivating this shift was the growing recognition of how many people died on the waiting list because the supply of kidneys was not adequate to meet the demand. These factors led to a new open-mindedness about the motivations of donors.

Aaron Spital, a nephrologist working at the University of Rochester School of Medicine in New York, did a series of surveys in the 1980s and 1990s showing how attitudes within the transplant community gradually shifted from almost universal rejection of stranger donors to their gradual acceptance. In 1987, about half of transplant centers would allow a friend to donate, while only 8 percent would allow strangers to donate (Spital 1994). Many centers reported that they had suspicions about the motivations of people who wanted to donate even though they had no emotional attachment to the recipient. The doctors worried that it would be morally wrong to allow someone to take the risk of donating a kidney to a stranger. By 1994, nearly twice as many centers (15 percent) accepted stranger donors. By 2000, the rate had more than doubled once more; 38 percent of the responding transplant centers would consider a donation from an altruistic stranger (Spital 2000).

Spital was fascinated by the struggles that nephrologists went through in trying to determine whether such altruists were noble or irrational. He cowrote a detailed report describing one such case (Spital and Levine 1998). A twenty-six-year-old woman had visited a transplant center and offered to donate a kidney to a young man she did not know. The young woman said she had heard about the man at her health club. She knew that many centers did not accept donations from strangers, so she claimed to be a friend of the young man's mother. She was interviewed and found to be rational and healthy. Eventually, the transplant center uncovered her initial deception and realized that she did not know the recipient. She was advised to meet with a psychiatrist.

The psychiatrist reported that she had no history of psychiatric illness or current psychological problems. She was married and had a six-month-old child at home. She had carefully thought about donating, discussed the decision with her family, and understood the risks. She described herself as "not very religious." During her upbringing, a high value was placed on helping others. The psychiatrist concluded that she was motivated by altruism and not at risk for psychiatric complications from donating. Nonetheless, the transplant committee remained troubled by what they perceived to be the impulsive nature of her decision. They recommended that the transplant be delayed for six months to give her time to reconsider. She did not change her mind and eventually donated.

This process would repeat itself time and again at different centers. A stranger would offer to donate. They would be referred for a psychological evaluation. Psychiatrists generally found that donors were psychologically healthy and understood the risks of the procedure.

In 2003, David Steinberg, director of the Section of Medical Ethics at the Lahey Clinic Medical Center in Burlington, Massachusetts, published a detailed description of one such psychological evaluation. A woman named Susan offered to donate a kidney to anybody who needed one. Steinberg was the psychologist who was consulted to evaluate her. His paper describes their encounter. Their exchange offers a unique glimpse into the motivations of an altruistic donor and into the forms of skepticism that doctors and psychologists bring to evaluations of such donors (Steinberg 2003).

Steinberg asked Susan why she would want to donate a kidney to a stranger. She replied, "I believe I should try to help people. This seems to be a perfect opportunity to help someone in a big way with minimal inconvenience to myself" (184). Steinberg pressed her on her characterization of the risks of surgery as a "minimal inconvenience." He told her that doctors estimated the mortality risk of donating at about 1/2500. Susan replied, "When I first thought about giving a kidney I was a bit freaked out thinking about the worst-case scenario—death or rejection by the other person of my kidney. I guess that's where my faith in God comes into it. I believe God wants me to use my life to help other people, and the rewards will be a much deeper happiness and a sense of real fulfillment in my life. Anyway, a one in 2,500 chance of death is a pretty slim one" (185).

"Most people who believe in God do not donate a kidney to a stranger," Steinberg told her.

"Just because 'most' people don't do it, isn't a reason to ban the minority who want to donate to a stranger" (185). She told him that she was a regular blood donor, had signed up to be a bone marrow donor, and now was willing to be a kidney donor. She saw these as all being logical actions for someone who wanted to show love to others.

"Did you consider that if anything went wrong, your seven-year-old son would not have a mother?" Steinberg asked (186).

Susan said that you could ask similar questions of police officers and firefighters. They could lose their lives. They choose to take a risk for the sake of the good that they are achieving through their dangerous occupations. We don't tell them that they shouldn't do their jobs. "Also, if I don't donate my kidney to someone, maybe their children will lose a parent or have a parent living on dialysis. The best I can do for my son as a mother is give him a good example. If I die, he will still have a loving, dedicated father, which is more than a lot of other children have" (187).

Susan felt that donating fit into her religious beliefs and was consistent with biblical injunctions to heal the sick. Steinberg worried that she was a member of a religious cult. Susan was offended by that and ended the interview by telling Steinberg, "You and other doctors have set yourselves up as judges of my motives with the possible intention of preventing hospitals from accepting the gift of my kidney" (187).

Susan's case raises interesting ethical considerations about the sorts of screening procedures that ought to be used to ascertain whether donors' motives are acceptable. One key element is that donation should be voluntary. Screening procedures look for evidence of coercion. But what counts as coercion? Religion can be a powerful motivator. But is such motivation coercive? Should we assume someone who is not very religious is acting freely and rationally while someone who is religious is not?

I thought of all this history as Martha was going through her painstaking evaluation process at the Mayo Clinic. In her decision to try to donate, she was unknowingly tiptoeing into a domain that existed only because some moral pioneers had challenged medical hierarchy. The thresholds of risk and the rules about donation have been constantly changing, challenged by both scientifically innovative doctors and by ethically innovative donors. Doctors eventually developed the rules and protocols in use today about who can or cannot be a donor, on the basis of assessments of the potential risk to the donor and the likelihood that the transplant will be successful. That is why Martha had to talk to the Mayo social worker. That is why she had to have her blood tested. That is why she had to be screened for medical and psychological problems.

Martha was frustrated by the bureaucratic hurdles she had to overcome to become an organ donor. But she was also relying on the doctors to protect her from her own impulses toward generosity. She counted on them to evaluate her risk level and not permit her to proceed if the risks were too high. She had hoped that donating would be easier. She certainly thought it should be faster. She was unaware of the history of stranger donors and of how her offer, while solicited, was nevertheless seen as controversial and ethically suspect. She thought the evaluation process was too cumbersome, time-consuming, and focused on irrelevant things.

And she was just getting started. I told her that it would have been much worse twenty years ago. Because she and Deb had no prior relationship, at many transplant centers she would not have been allowed to donate at all.

7

What Are the Risks?

(MARTHA)

Dr. Bentall next reviewed the risks, both surgical and medical, to donating a kidney. He was impressed that I had read the recent study that my primary care doctor had provided. He confirmed my understanding of the study, including the limitations to the data. He said there were also studies that showed there were long-term positive psychological impacts for living organ donors. Many said it brought greater meaning to their own lives.

Now Dr. Bentall turned to Don. How did he feel about my donating a kidney?

"Martha always needs a project," Don replied. "This seems like a good one."

I was touched at how well Don knew me. We had never talked about this adventure in those terms, but he was absolutely right. I always needed a project. And I had latched onto this one.

Dr. Bentall was amused. He nodded with a smile.

Then he turned to the screen to review my numbers. With two exceptions, he reported, all the tests looked good. My creatinine level, an important marker for kidney function, was normal. So was my urine. Most of my other blood tests were good too. I did not have anemia, HIV, hepatitis, syphilis, or tuberculosis.

There are two potential issues, he said. My smile froze. That did not sound good. My weight insecurities aside, I had basically been approaching these evaluations like all the other tests in my privileged, high-performing life—I secretly assumed I would ace them. Now the doctor was telling me I had less-than-perfect scores on two midterm quizzes. Did this mean my final grade was at risk?

Dr. Bentall did not bring up my weight directly. He was concerned about my fasting glucose level. At 110, it was in the prediabetes range and ten points higher than the maximum level acceptable for a kidney donor. Since my history of gestational diabetes was also correlated with a long-term risk of adult onset diabetes, this was of particular concern.

The high level made no sense to me. My glucose levels had been normal during my annual physicals. And Mayo's hemoglobin A1C number—which measures average blood glucose levels over the past three months—was also normal. Wasn't that countervailing evidence that I was doing okay on the blood sugar front? Dr. Bentall agreed that this one blood sample, taken after a full day of travel and my irregular eating while on the road, might not be reflecting true risk. But the Transplant Selection Committee would always err on the side of caution for a living donor.

Since the evidence was inconclusive, would it make sense to retest? I asked.

Dr. Bentall thought it would, and that we should do the more definitive glucose tolerance test. That test should tell us a lot more, he said.

The second issue Dr. Bentall brought up was my blood pressure. While I usually tested on the high side of normal, my blood pressure readings in his office that day (five in a row, taken by an automatic monitor at two-minute intervals) were high. That did not surprise me—I felt like I had been extremely stressed since I got to Rochester. When I suggested that possibility, Dr. Bentall concurred. Yes, that can happen here, the nephrologist said. This is a pretty stressful routine. That is why we do the eighteen-hour continuous blood pressure test. Those results will tell us a lot more.

What about my age? I asked. Did that pose a health risk to me as a donor? Not if everything else lines up, Dr. Bentall said. In fact, there were advantages to being an older donor. For one thing, if I had already made it to sixty-one without developing kidney disease, hypertension, or diabetes, I was probably in good shape to live out my natural life with a single kidney. And I did not have to worry about a lone kidney keeping me healthy as long as a younger donor would. A thirty-year-old kidney donor had a lot more years to go than I did.

Dr. Bentall also explained that one of the few nonmedical risks of living with only one kidney was organ damage from contact sports. I assured him that my contact sports days were over.

Finally, he said, while this was not a significant issue, some younger female donors express concern about the stress that pregnancy can put on a single kidney. Just to confirm, he smiled, you aren't planning on becoming pregnant again, are you? Those days are over too, I said.

I had conflicting feelings about Dr. Bentall's caution regarding my blood glucose and blood pressure results. On the one hand, they did not seem like significant deviations, and I was inclined to overlook them and get on with the donation. On the other hand, I did not want to rush into a completely voluntary procedure that would cause me serious health problems down the road.

I had made that mistake once before, and I was still paying for it. Eighteen years earlier, I had impulsively agreed to a Lasik procedure in the hope of "throwing away my glasses for good." The eye surgeon had been eager to operate. I had gone to his office for an evaluation for the corrective procedure. After a cursory exam, he declared me a good candidate for Lasik. He said he would be happy to help me, and after the surgery he would be pleased to have my endorsement to my wide circle of personal and professional connections.

After the encouragement and the flattery, he pulled a famous sales trick, looking at his schedule and announcing, "I just had a cancellation for three days from now. If you want the slot, I can get you in right away. Otherwise you'll have to wait a few months for an appointment." I took the bait and took the appointment.

I ended up having Lasik three days later without getting a second opinion and without doing any research. Only much later did I learn that my surgeon, eager to add me to his list of successful patients, had neglected to perform one of the most important tests available to evaluate someone for that procedure—a test for dry eyes.

As it turned out, I most likely had an underlying dry eye malady, and the procedure left me with severe, chronic dry eyes. The condition makes me miserable to this day. My eyes are constantly irritated, scratchy, and painful, making it difficult to drive and almost impossible to read for any length of time.

I tried every remedy anyone recommended. Nothing helped. I finally became resigned to living with the discomfort, settling on a brand of artificial tears that seemed to help the most, as long as I used them every fifteen to twenty minutes. For the past eighteen years, I had literally never gone anywhere without a bottle of eye drops. I use eye drops when I work, when I eat, when I talk on the phone, when I am in meetings, when I read, write, drive, go to movies, exercise. I use them when I wake up in the middle of the night to pee. Sometimes I use them during sex.

So I knew what it meant to rush into an elective surgery and have it go terribly wrong.

Now I had to honestly face the question: Were these test results signaling I might be doing it again? Was I letting my enthusiasm override reasonable caution? Was I pushing too hard to do this? Was I rushing into another mistake?

The biggest medical risk for kidney donors is the chance of end stage renal disease later in life. Diabetes and hypertension (high blood pressure), are two major contributors. If the tests showed I had high blood pressure or increased risk for diabetes, then maybe I was not cut out to be a donor. I might have to choose my health over Deb's.

And we still had two more days of testing before we would have any definitive results.

Meeting My Surgeon

The next day, my second at Mayo, began with one of the most important tests, an abdominal CT scan. This time the trick was not to pee on command; it was not to pee. I was instructed to drink half a bottle of water (no soda alternative for this one), and then sit in the waiting room while my bladder started to fill. About fifteen minutes later I was called back to the CT scan room, where the tech strapped a contraption around my waist that resembled a weight belt with deflated balloon-type things located on either side about where my kidneys were. They took several abdominal images like that, then inflated the "balloons" to put pressure on my abdomen. I did not really have to pee yet, but I could see the pressure might get me there pretty quickly. Then the tech injected contrast dye into a vein on the inside of my forearm. It did not hurt, but the sudden warmth of the dye spreading downward was disconcerting. I was relatively sure I had not wet myself on the exam table, but that rapid flush made it hard to be certain. A few more scans, and I was out and up—and relieved to find myself perfectly dry. None of this hurt. But it was all pretty weird.

Several hours later, I met my first Mayo transplant surgeon. After a brief greeting, he pulled up my CT scans on his computer screen, while I viewed them on my phone. "You have textbook perfect kidneys," he said admiringly. Pointing to the scans, he showed me how blood flows from the abdominal aorta into each kidney via the left and right renal arteries. One of those renal arteries would be severed to remove a kidney for transplantation. Over time most people grow "extra" veins from their kidneys back to the abdominal aorta, like a tree growing new branches. These extra channels are not important in healthy people: they do not serve any vital function and they do not cause problems. But they can make removing a kidney more difficult, causing the surgery to take longer and creating more opportunity for bleeding. Astoundingly, my kidneys had behaved; they had grown no such extra appendages. They were perfect.

I was liking this exam a lot. Finally, someone was giving me an A+. I have great kidneys, I thought smugly. So there!

Like everyone at Mayo, the surgeon was extremely self-confident. "This is a simple surgery, it only takes about ninety minutes—I do several every week," he said with great assurance. "Mayo has never lost a living kidney donor, and we have never had a significant postsurgical complication." Others had told me that the surgery would actually take two to three hours. What the cavalier surgeon meant was that his part would only take ninety minutes. The anesthesia, prep, and closing—all parts that belonged to someone else—would take another thirty to ninety minutes. He was thinking of his time, not mine.

I was also realizing that the surgery was the least risky part of donating a kidney.

The more significant risk to the donor is the less dramatic lifetime risk of living with only one kidney. I realized I should be grateful for Mayo's careful screening. It was increasingly clear they would approve me to donate only if they felt that my lifetime risks were very low.

As our consultation concluded, the surgeon repeated the litany I had now heard many times: "This is surgery you do not need. Your recipient has other options. You may tell anyone at any time up until you are wheeled into surgery that you want out—all the recipient will be told is that there is a medical concern about the procedure. Do you still want to go forward with the donation?" I nodded for the umpteenth time. I was going to trust Mayo's rigorous evaluation process. If I was accepted after all these tests, then I was still in. I had not come this far to back out now.

Psychosocial Issues

The nonmedical consultations were not uncomfortable or difficult, though they added to my mounting fatigue as the days wore on.

The financial counselor was in charge of making sure I understood the financial ramifications of donating a kidney. My recipient's insurance would pay for my donor evaluation, surgery, and all postoperative and follow-up care, including my hospital stay, outpatient consultations and procedures, tests, and medications. Nonetheless, there would be significant out-of-pocket costs that would fall to us, primarily related to travel and missed work. There was some financial aid available for donors in need, including the National Living Donor Assistance Center, an agency funded by the federal Department of Health and Human Services, which assists with travel costs for donors. However, as the center's website notes, they only pay for "travel, lodging, meals, and incidental expenses," not lost wages or childcare.

The criteria to qualify for this type of help are tight—both the donor and recipient must earn less than three times the poverty level. In 2016, less than 9 percent of living donors got support from the center. I did not qualify.

There were also other ways to limit the out-of-pocket burden on donors and their families. The financial counselor told us about the nearby Gift of Life Transplant House that offered accommodation at very low rates—thirty dollars per night and an additional one-time fee of forty dollars for room cleaning. She also explained that my home state of Kansas is one of a handful of states that allows income tax deductions (up to $5,000) for living organ donors' unreimbursed travel, lodging, and medical expenses.

I do not know why the Mayo financial counselor did not mention it, but I later learned that Deb's insurance carrier, UnitedHealthcare, the largest insurer in the country, had recently announced that it would reimburse travel and lodging expenses for all kidney donors and their companions whose intended transplant recipients were insured by the company. According to the company website, the reimbursement, up to $5,000, would include the donor's initial evaluation, the transplant surgery, and follow-up evaluations up to two years after the donation.

Though some of these benefits might help defray the costs of donating an organ, it was obvious that being an out-of-town living organ donor is expensive. Our out-of-pocket expenses were already adding up (three nights in the Rochester hotel, meals, and mileage to and from Kansas City), as well as Don using a week of his annual paid time off. The financial counselor wanted to be sure I understood this would likely cost a lot more money and take a lot more time if we proceeded with the surgery.

Was any of this going to be an obstacle?

I explained that Don and I could afford the travel expenses, and we were empty nesters, so we would not need to pay for childcare while we were away from home. Unlike so many who might otherwise be willing and able to donate organs, Don and I were in a financial position to make money a nonissue.

As for time off work, I was now retired, and Don had enough paid time off to use for our trips to Minnesota. Once again, we were in a very fortunate position. But thinking about the issues got me thinking about all the people who might want to donate but for whom the financial barriers were just too high. I began to wonder whether there might be a better way to deal with the many hidden costs of donation. If, as a nation, we really wanted to address the undersupply of organs for transplant, we would need to think creatively and proactively address some of the many barriers that make it difficult or impossible for people to donate.

A Possible Glitch?

Since our lunch in Kansas City, Deb and I had stayed in regular communication. We texted often and talked on the phone when the mood struck us or we had some pressing logistical issue to work through. On my second day at Mayo, Deb texted and asked me to call; something important had come up. Her nurse transplant coordinator had called to tell her that when they ran my fresh blood against her stored blood they got a concerning result about our histocompatibility. Deb was supposed to send more blood up to Mayo to rerun the tests the following week. In the meantime, she hoped I might get more information from the doctors while I was there.

Nobody had mentioned anything about incompatibility to me, but I had received a call from the Mayo lab on my cell phone the day before asking me to return to have more blood drawn before the end of the day. The lab tech said she did not know why I had been called back, but she thought maybe one of my earlier samples had been tainted somehow, and they were drawing a replacement as a precaution. At the time that had seemed like an unlikely explanation, since Dr. Bentall had already reviewed all my lab results. He had not suggested anything was missing. But no one offered a better explanation, and I was so overwhelmed managing the exhausting evaluation schedule that I forgot about the second lab draw until Deb called. Even with the information she provided, there was not much to be done. I did my best not to worry about this added complication while we pushed through the remaining appointments.

Donor Education

A highlight in the middle of the long appointment slog was the donor education class, which involved a meeting with other potential kidney donors, recipients, and caregivers who were also at Mayo for evaluation.

Up until this point I had only known a few people who had actually given away a kidney. One was Cheryl, the family friend from Omaha who saved my cousin Ann. I also had the opportunity to have lunch with Judy, a Kansas City attorney who had donated a kidney to her mother many years before. Another was Aaron, a good friend from our Kansas City synagogue, who had donated a kidney to a fellow congregant in his new synagogue in Philadelphia in 2017. In an interview in the Philadelphia newspaper *Jewish Exponent*, Aaron credited the inspiration for his mitzvah to Rabbi Shmuly Yanklowitz, whom we knew from his time in Kansas City years before. An article in the *Times of Israel* recounted how

Shmuly had read about a fifteen-year-old Israeli boy who needed a kidney and volunteered to donate. All the donors I talked to felt the entire process had been manageable and meaningful. None expressed regrets.

The other potential donors and recipients in the donor education class seemed like perfectly reasonable people, embarking on a perfectly reasonable quest. Still, I was the only potential donor seeking to give to someone who had been a complete stranger. Even though we were all lining up for the same medical procedure, mine was a more unusual case.

One mother-daughter pair caught my attention. The young adult daughter was being assessed as a potential donor, and the mom told the group she had donated a kidney about a decade before. Later, I ran into the mom in the waiting room of the Transplant Center. She was very friendly, and I asked if she would mind sharing more about her story. She explained that her older daughter had been born with serious kidney problems as well as other medical issues, and a number of years ago the mom had successfully donated a kidney. Now that kidney was failing, and the daughter needed another transplant. Her father, this woman's husband, had low kidney function and could not donate. The younger sister, who I had just met in class, was the only sibling. She matched.

My heart went out to this mother. The daughter who was here to be tested was a recent college graduate and freshly married with a new job, the mother told me; she hoped to start a family in a few years. But she also wanted to help her sister if she could. The mom was determined to stay objective and let this young woman make her own choice without judgment or pressure. But I could imagine how difficult this must be.

I wanted Mayo to approve me to donate. But if they did not, I was not facing the loss of a child. I thought about how being a "stranger donor" might actually be easier than matching to donate to a family member.

The nurse who led the donor education class described the procedure in detail—two small inch-long incisions for the instruments, then the larger incision for the sleeve that would accommodate the surgeon's hand for the all-important organ retrieval. She pointed to a door at the end of the hall leading to Charlton 9. "That's the hospital wing, right there. Through those doors is the transplant floor."

The nurse explained that admission was on the first floor and pre-op right below that. "We'll put in an IV, put in a catheter, and you'll be good to go." She made it sound so simple.

Then she gave the donor protection speech once again: "This is surgery you do not need. Your recipient has other options. You may tell anyone at any time up until you are wheeled into surgery that you want out—all the recipient will be told is that you are medically unable to donate."

The nurse then said she was going to play a video showing the surgical procedure. Anyone should feel free to be excused at this point. Everyone else stayed, but I grabbed Don's hand and steered us out of the room. I am not generally squeamish, but this did not seem like a good time to take chances.

Did They Think I Was Irrational?

I also had appointments with Lisa, my nurse transplant coordinator; Margo, my designated donor advocate; and a social worker who was assigned to assess my mental fitness as an organ donor.

Lisa and I had been communicating by phone and by email for several months now, so it was a pleasure to finally meet her in person. We talked about the process and what else I could expect

during my remaining time at Mayo. I asked about the blood compatibility issues Deb had called about. Had Lisa heard anything?
No, she had not. Her best advice was to talk to Dr. Bentall during
my wrap-up appointment at the end of my three-day visit. Maybe
he would know more.

Margo was warm and friendly. She explained it was her job
to look out for my best interests throughout the process. I com-
plained mildly about having to return for the substance abuse
evaluation and asked if there was anything she could do about
that. She was sympathetic, but did not have much to offer in the
way of a solution.

By the time I met with the second social worker, I was starting
to lose it. The young woman was sweet and had a solid mastery of
the questions printed in front of her, even if she did insist on using
my name in every other sentence in that annoying way common
to insurance salespeople and preschool teachers. Plowing through
the required questions, her tone fell somewhere between boredom
and false cheer.

Was anyone paying me to do this? No. Why did I want to do it?
I had a cousin who received a kidney transplant, so it felt like the
right thing to do. Had I had any life experiences that made me
sad? Yes—when my mother died I was very sad. If my recipient
did not fare well after the surgery, how did I think I would feel?
Very, very sad.

Did I have any concerns? YES. I let my carefully controlled
façade drop. I have a big concern.

"I do not have a substance abuse problem. I worked in the field
of child abuse and neglect. I know what a drug problem looks like.
I do not have a drug problem. I smoked some pot on vacation in
Colorado, and I disclosed that on my initial questionnaire. Drug
addicts would never disclose that. You have checked my blood and

my urine; there has been no indication of drug use of any kind. You have asked me to submit to a substance abuse evaluation, and I have agreed. However, you cannot find me an appointment while I am here. I have checked for cancelations throughout my visit this week—to no avail. I have offered to stay in Rochester an extra day. I have offered to do this in person in Kansas City and fax you the results. None of these options works for you. So I have to take two more days out of my schedule to fly back here, rent a car, spend the night in a hotel, report for an early morning appointment—the only one you have available—and then fly home again. Everyone keeps saying that living organ donation is 'scheduled at the convenience of the donor.' This is not convenient."

The young woman gave me a mildly consoling and infuriatingly noncommittal look. "I understand that you're upset about this." Great, I thought. No help from that quarter. Now they will probably decide I am not only a drug addict, but I have anger management issues too.

But I had underestimated this young professional. Two hours later, my cell phone rang. It was the social worker. "I talked to others on the transplant team and we have all agreed that the cannabis use is not an issue. I have canceled your substance abuse evaluation in April; you do not have to return for that appointment." I could have jumped through the phone and hugged her. If I were still running my nonprofit, I would have hired her.

8

Unnecessary Bureaucratic Barriers or Appropriate Patient Protection?

(JOHN)

Transplant centers have very strong motivations to encourage people to become living kidney donors. Each donation saves the lives of patients on the transplant waiting list. Furthermore, as waiting lists get longer, and people spend more time on dialysis, they become sicker. On average, transplant recipients today are older and sicker than they used to be. In 2002, the average age of transplant recipients was fifty-one. Ten years later, it was fifty-five (Axelrod et al. 2017). This leads to more surgical and postsurgical complications when an organ finally becomes available and higher expenses to provide care for transplant recipients. Reimbursement rates have not kept up with these increases. Thus, in addition to improving patient outcomes, hospitals have a financial incentive to help kidney patients get transplants as soon as possible. Transplants performed earlier in the course of a patient's disease are good for recipients and good for medical centers.

But transplant centers also have strong motivations to screen donors and to not accept people who are not physically and psychologically healthy. They want donors who are physically healthy, both in order to be sure that their donated kidney is healthy and to make sure that they are not harmed by either the operation or, in the long term, by having only one kidney. And they want donors who are psychologically healthy, and thus competent to make this very serious decision, and without suffering undue mental distress after the procedure.

Of course, even with the most careful screening, donation still has risks. All operations have risks. The National Kidney Foundation warns potential donors on its website that they could suffer a long list of complications as a result of the surgery ("Risks of Surgery" n.d.). These complications include pain, life-threatening postoperative infections, blood clots and strokes, urinary tract infections, and allergic reactions to anesthesia or other drugs. They cite a mortality rate from donation of 0.03 percent—three deaths for every ten thousand donations. That means that, in the United States, one or two donors will die from donation every year. Major complications occur after about 5 percent of operations. Minor complications occur after 20 percent (Lentine and Patel 2012).

Donors are more likely than nondonors with similar characteristics to develop hypertension (Boudville et al. 2006; Garg et al. 2008). Hypertension can cause kidney failure. Some kidney donors have developed kidney failure and required a transplant themselves (Gibney et al. 2007). The risks of postdonation hypertension are higher among donors who are African American or Hispanic (Lentine et al. 2010). Should they be denied the opportunity to donate, using the exact same criteria that are used for Caucasian donors? If so, then because of histocompatibility issues, there will be fewer transplants from biological relatives for African American and Hispanic patients who need a kidney. The most cautious use of kidneys might lead to systematic discrimination against minorities. Their overall health care costs will be higher and their outcomes worse. To loosen the criteria, however, could mean that more minority donors would go on to have lifelong health problems. Either choice could exacerbate existing disparities.

As science improves, we may be able to refine our prognostic tools and give each donor an estimate of their own personalized risk factors and likely outcomes, based on their specific health data, demographic information, and studies of predictive genetic markers. As in Martha's tale, somebody would have to weigh those health risks against the patient's own desires and against the data showing that donors report improved psychosocial well-being and feel that that their own quality of life is better than it was before they donated. They also score higher on such measures than non-donors (Lentine, Lam, and Segev 2019).

So donation could be bad for the body but good for the soul. How should clinicians balance those competing claims?

Many potential donors express frustration with the lengthy, inconvenient evaluation process that Martha described. One felt moved to post a lament on the kidney transplant forum on the DaVita Kidney Care website: "For all the people out there waiting for a donor, I hope you know that there are people wanting to donate. I have been trying for months to get the donation process going . . . I think people wanting to donate probably just give up after a while." Such sentiments also show up in studies of potential donors. One series of focus groups that included people who were knowledgeable and supportive of donation probed the reasons participants did not actually donate. One said, "I wish the process could be quicker, there are people dying and it shouldn't take so long to get checked out as a donor" (Dorflinger et al. 2018, 33).

One-Day Evaluations

These frustrating barriers to donation can be overcome if our medical system chooses to be innovative. With focus and determination, it is possible to design a program to evaluate donors more quickly and efficiently. Belfast City Hospital in Ireland recently instituted a one-day evaluation (Graham and Courtney 2018). This was a major effort that required collaboration between multiple specialties, including radiology, histocompatibility and immunogenetics, nuclear medicine, and cardiac investigations, along with reorganization of the local transplantation service. Over five years, they evaluated 431 potential donors. Of these, 284 (66 percent) went on to donate, and 48 (11 percent) were deemed unsuitable for medical reasons. Another 18 (4 percent) withdrew themselves from consideration. Overall donation rates rose from just four per one million people in the population to thirty-three per one million people. Donors' perceptions of the process also improved dramatically.

Fifty people who proceeded to donation in Belfast in 2011 were surveyed, forty-nine of whom responded. Of the sixteen assessed before the one-day evaluation was instituted, 38 percent rated the process as "poor" or "very poor," and a further 25 percent gave a "neutral" score with comments such as "the whole process took 18 months" and "had to wait 8–10 weeks for each result and then another 8–10 weeks for the next test appointment. Very frustrating!"

Of the thirty-three who had the one-day assessment, 94 percent rated it as "very good," and the rest, as "good," with examples of narrative being "it was excellent that all the appointments were on the same day in the same hospital" and "a day assessment suited me because of work" (Graham and Courtney 2018, 211–12).

It is surprising, given the success of this program, that transplant centers in the United States have not tested a similar approach. Such endeavors might well increase the efficiency of donor evaluation, decrease wait times, and ultimately increase the number of donors without sacrificing the benefits that come with careful and rigorous screening. Belfast City Hospital has shown how we can increase efficiency and patient satisfaction without sacrificing safety. It just takes a shift in the ethos of the institution.

9

The Endgame

(MARTHA)

My meeting with the hypertension counselor went well, and I began to feel better about that issue. Although my eighteen-hour blood pressure test showed elevated readings while I was running around Mayo, it smoothed out as soon as I left the clinic for the day. The tech told me he was not the decision maker on my donor status, but overall, he thought the test results looked good. If it were up to him, he said, I would be approved. He advised me to monitor my salt intake. Other than that, he thought I was fine.

The results of my glucose tolerance test were equally encouraging. My blood sugar level two hours after swallowing the sugary gunk required for the test was 110. Anything lower than 140 is normal. Consistent with my hemoglobin A1C readings and my annual glucose tests, my body was processing blood sugar just fine.

Finally, three long days after I first entered the Mayo Clinic, I walked into my final meeting with Dr. Bentall. I was completely depleted, fueled solely by determination and hope. I had toughed out three days of grueling tests, gotten mostly good news along the way, retested where necessary, and was now ready to be rewarded for my efforts with a very big "Atta girl." I was ready to be done.

Dr. Bentall walked in, as warm and engaging as before. The results are good, he said, but not perfect. We have some decisions to make.

My heart sank. After all this time and trouble, I thought, please don't let him say no.

The best news was first. I passed the psychological screening with flying colors. I had an excellent psychosocial support system and enough money. Dr. Bentall was amused that I had talked my way out of returning for the substance abuse evaluation. "You must have been very persuasive," he said.

My kidney function was excellent, my EKG and chest X-ray were normal, and the surgeon reported no issues from his review of my kidney scans and his examination of my abdomen and lungs. The more rigorous, second glucose test revealed that my blood sugar was not a problem.

The only remaining issue was my blood pressure: 63 percent of my diastolic readings while awake were over 80, and 46 percent of my systolic readings while awake were over 130. Too high.

I was pretty stressed here, I said cautiously.

Dr. Bentall nodded. But I bet your real life back home actually includes some stress too, he suggested wryly. He had me there.

If I were just a regular patient seeking a hypertension consultation, he would not be worried, Dr. Bentall explained. But I was a potential kidney donor, seeking to have surgery I did not need that would leave me with only one kidney for the rest of my life. That raised the bar.

He outlined four available choices: I could end the process now. I could lose some weight and reduce salt intake and retest in a few months. I could start on a very low dose of antihypertensive medication and retest in two weeks. Or he could take my file with the current results to the Transplant Selection Committee and hope for the best.

I could tell he was not excited about the last option. I was not going to take the first option; I was definitely not going to quit after all we had just gone through. And I was definitely not going to stake Deb's life on my ability to successfully lose weight within a short period of time. That sounded like hell on earth to my fat-shamed soul.

That left door number three: start on blood pressure meds and retest. I'm inclined toward that option, I told the doctor. What are the side effects to this medication?

Most people report no side effects at all, Dr. Bentall told me. A low percentage report a dry cough. It is a well-tolerated medication, even at much higher doses than you will be taking.

What about the retest? I asked.

You can do that at home, he explained. Mayo would have the blood pressure monitor mailed to Kansas City, I would wear it for eighteen hours, then ship it back to the provider to read the results.

And we can do this all in two weeks? Yes.

And if it works, then we're good to go to the committee? Yes.

You do not have to do this at all, Dr. Bentall reminded me again.

Actually, I said, I think I do.

This had become more than a chance to save Deb. Weirdly, this had also become a referendum on my body. I was determined to pass.

He nodded and typed on his keyboard. The blood pressure medication, Lisinopril, would be waiting at my pharmacy in Kansas City when we got home.

This will work, he said, confidently. I really do not see any barriers to your donating a kidney. You are a good candidate. Actually, better than most.

Finally, the reassurance I had been hoping for.

What about the recent concern over my blood match with Deb? I asked. Dr. Bentall did not know anything about that. Because of the firewall between my care team and Deb's care team, he did not even know her name, let alone have access to her medical records. I had more information than he had.

He said it sounded like there might be an issue with the crossmatch results. Different from tissue typing, the crossmatch tests are one more way to help ensure a recipient will not reject their new kidney. It is rare, but even an infection or a bug bite can cause a change in the antibodies of either the donor or the recipient after the initial tests. Dr. Bentall said I would have to wait for more information from Deb's care team, presumably delivered via Deb after the new blood tests were run.

In the meantime, he said, I could think about a plan B. If the new blood tests ruled me out to donate directly to Deb, would I be willing to be part of Mayo's Kidney Paired Donation program instead? I had read about kidney donor chains online. These more complicated arrangements involved someone like me donating a kidney to a person who had a relative or friend who wanted to donate but was not a match. That person would get my kidney and then "their" donor would donate to someone else who had a relative or friend who wanted to donate but was not a match. And so on. Sometimes these were just four-way matches or "pairs," but some of the chains were very long—involving ten or more people. The longest known chain, which was still ongoing at the University of Alabama at Birmingham's School of Medicine, was approaching one hundred participants, according to their website (Pope 2018).

Of course I would be willing to participate in a chain, I told him. From my point of view, the risks and benefits were identical: I would give away my kidney. Deb would get a kidney. If what happened in between was more complex than we originally envisioned, I did not see why that should make any difference. In fact, if participating in a chain resulted in even more people getting help, then it seemed like an even better idea.

By the time Don and I left Rochester that afternoon, my head was spinning. This was not the unambiguous success I had imagined before coming up to Mayo. I had pictured driving home in triumph, calling Deb, and then announcing to my friends and family that I was approved to donate. While I had escaped returning to Mayo for the substance abuse evaluation, there was still going to be a delay while we reran the blood pressure test and reran the blood match. We were not done yet.

Don and I planned to spend that night in a hotel in downtown Minneapolis and then meet up with our son the following evening for the first night of Passover. We drove the ninety-minute trip in a stupor, stopping for a meal I could barely eat. Finally, we got up to our hotel room and, overwhelmed and exhausted, I slept for twelve hours straight.

10

Paired Exchanges, Chain Donations, and Organ Markets

(JOHN)

Most people who donate kidneys choose to donate to a specific recipient. Even if it is not a relative or somebody they know, it may be somebody from their community or someone with whom they feel a connection. Like Martha and Deb, they might not know each other initially, but their relationship grows during the lengthy donation process. One limitation to such "directed" donations is that, often, prospective donors are not well-matched with specific recipients. In fact, the odds of such a match are statistically very far-fetched. One way to encourage donations even when there is no match is to use an innovation called "paired exchange." This is the plan B that the Mayo nephrologist had mentioned to Martha.

The idea of paired donation exchange is conceptually simple. Imagine that somebody (call them "donor 1") wants to donate a kidney to a specific person ("recipient 1"), but is histologically incompatible with the intended recipient. Imagine that, at the same time, there was a similar poorly matched donor-recipient pair at another hospital. Then imagine that donor 1 was histocompatible with recipient 2 and donor 2 with recipient 1. Instead of the donors donating to their own intended recipients, each would donate to the other. From the donors' perspective, the risks were the same. From the recipients' perspective, outcomes would be much better as a result of receiving a histocompatible organ than they would be if they received their own designated recipient's organ. Figure 1 is a graphic showing how it works.

This seems like a great way to increase the supply of organs for transplant. But, when first proposed, it raised some legal questions. At that time, the National Organ Transplant Act (1984) was the prevailing law in the United States. It prohibited the "commercial exchange" of organs. The law characterized commercial exchange as "transfer [of a] human organ for valuable consideration." Lawyers wondered whether a paired kidney exchange was a sort of barter and thus the beginning of a gray market in organs.

Writing in the *New England Journal of Medicine*, Lainie Friedman Ross, a physician and bioethicist at the University of Chicago, joined colleagues in arguing that paired exchanges should not be considered as commercial exchanges. They noted that the intent of the law prohibiting commercial exchange was to "prevent the exploitation of living persons who might be willing to sell their body parts for profit" (Ross et al. 1997, 1753). Paired exchanges, by contrast, enlist altruistic donors who, because of medical criteria (organ incompatibility), cannot donate directly to the intended recipients but are willing to make donations that will benefit their loved ones indirectly (Ross et al. 1997). Eventually, the federal law

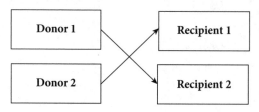

FIGURE 1
Paired exchange

governing organ selling was amended to explicitly permit "human organ paired donation" (Marshall 2007).

Then things got more complicated. Some suggested that, instead of a simple paired exchange of kidneys, one could create a serial chain of donor-recipient pairs, so that donor 1 gave to recipient 2, donor 2 to recipient 3, and so on. Such an arrangement might look something like figure 2.

A further expansion of this practice took place in 2017, with the world's first kidney-liver swap. A woman needed a kidney, and her daughter was a match, but the daughter was not a good donor candidate because she was at risk for the same hereditary kidney disease. But she did have a healthy liver. Meanwhile, another patient needed a liver transplant, and her sister was willing to be a living

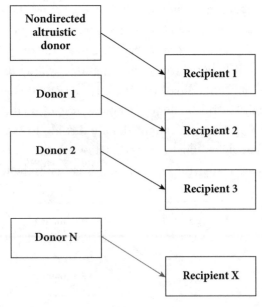

FIGURE 2
Chain exchange

liver donor. But her liver was too small for the procedure. Doctors at the University of California Medical Center in San Francisco paired the two families; patient 1's daughter donated a portion of her liver to patient 2, and patient 2's sister donated a kidney to patient 1. The university's ethics committee debated whether this exchange was ethical, since the risk of donating a portion of a liver was so much greater than the risk of donating a kidney.

Ultimately, they approved the transplants, and that paired donation took place (Torres et al. 2019).

11

The Odyssey Continues

(MARTHA)

I came home from Minneapolis determined to put a good face on our evaluation trip to Mayo. "We are very close," I told the friends who knew what I was trying to do. "Just a few more hurdles."

A week later I got heartening news. Deb called from Florida with a jubilant voice. "It's okay. We're still a match." No one had offered any explanation for the intermediate glitch. All she had been told was that I was still designated as her match, and that we were waiting for my case to go before the Transplant Selection Committee to learn whether I was approved to donate.

But as soon as that obstacle fell, a new one appeared in its place. Don and I had picked up the prescription for Lisinopril, my new hypertension medication, at our local CVS on the drive home from Minneapolis, and I had started taking the pills the following day. Dr. Bentall had said I should give the medication two weeks to take effect before redoing the eighteen-hour blood pressure test. Looking at my calendar, I had decided Monday, April 16—two weeks and two days after I started the drug—would be a good day to stay home and get that done. Unfortunately, someone at Mayo jumped the gun, and the blood pressure cuff arrived on my doorstep on April 3. I called the 800 number for First Medical in Nebraska that was listed on the accompanying instruction sheet to see whether it would cause a problem to just hold the cuff until I was ready for the test. The customer service rep was courteous, but firm. Yes, it was a big problem. The battery in the monitor wouldn't last more than a week, and my results might fail to record. I should send the cuff back and call when I wanted them to resend. I dutifully stuffed the blood pressure apparatus back in its case and took the package to FedEx to return. Another Mayo hiccup. From the start, I had followed every instruction with meticulous care. It made me nervous that they could not do the same.

Dr. Bentall told me that about 30 percent of patients who took Lisinopril reported a persistent dry cough. I turned out to be one of them. Within a few days of starting the medication, I was coughing all the time, day and night. I had to leave three movies and a play midshow so I would not annoy the other patrons. Cough medicines did not help. Warm beverages did not help. Liquor did not help. The only thing that helped was sucking on menthol lozenges, which I started to do constantly, even while trying to fall asleep. I suspected that was a choking risk, though I was too miserable to care.

I was going to have to stop the Lisinopril. And then what? Would my unmedicated blood pressure disqualify me from donating?

Don, less anxious and more rational, encouraged me to call my primary care physician. He recommended switching to a low dose of Losartan; he would write a prescription for me to fill right away. I was greatly relieved. But I did not want to mess with anything before the next blood pressure test. Bolstered by the knowledge that the end was in sight, I stuck with the Lisinopril for another week, coughing furiously while I waited to retest my blood pressure.

On April 12, a second blood pressure cuff arrived from the provider in Nebraska, this time right on schedule. I spent April 16 hanging out at home, coughing, and watching the cuff inflate and

deflate at regular intervals. I also used the Mayo portal to confer with Lisa, my nurse transplant coordinator, about the cough
and my doctor's recommendation to switch to Losartan. The next
message I got via the portal was from Dr. Bentall: "Hi, Ms. Gershun. Yes, a recognized side-effect. Happy for the switch. Thanks
for checking."

The next morning, I switched to the new medicine, packed up
the blood pressure kit, and took it to FedEx to return to Nebraska.
Two days later, Lisa called from Mayo to say the eighteen-hour
readings looked good. Maybe my decision to stick with the Lisinopril through the test had been unnecessarily draconian. But it had
worked—my blood pressure now met Mayo standards!

Lisa also said she was preparing the file to take my case to the
Selection Committee the following week. She noticed they were
still missing the PAP smear, colonoscopy, and mammogram
results from my Kansas City providers. Could I please have them
faxed over right away?

I was taken aback. What did she mean "missing"? I had spent
countless weeks conferring with Mayo about the requirements
for this kidney donation and three days practically living at their
clinic. During all that time, not a single person had mentioned
sending these test results.

Now the deadline was imminent. In order to take my case to the
committee the following week, Lisa needed my test results right
away. Another screw-up from the famous Mayo Clinic, and once
again, I was paying the price. They were making it really hard to
donate my kidney.

This time the solution was simple brute force. I canceled my
plans for the afternoon and spent the rest of the day calling various medical providers to get my records. My ob-gyn had my PAP
smear, the breast imaging center at the local hospital had my

mammogram, and, thankfully, my primary care doctor had my colonoscopy results. I was able to download my mammogram from the hospital's secure portal and fax it to Mayo, and my doctor's office faxed my colonoscopy results directly. The receptionist at my ob-gyn insisted I drive to the office and pick up a hard copy of my mammogram results. Once again I wondered how a potential donor in a different life situation would have managed this.

Lisa used exclamation points when she emailed to let me know that my file was complete. But then casually informed me that, oh, by the way, the Selection Committee meeting was being postponed a week. I need not have rushed at all.

I spent the following week trying to think about other things and managing to think about nothing else. My cough persisted, a constant reminder that I was waiting to hear from Mayo. Finally, on Thursday morning, April 26, my phone buzzed: 507. I stepped away to answer. It was Lisa. "You're good to go!"

I pulled up the notes that were loaded into my Mayo portal:

Results of committee deliberation

Patient was presented today, Thursday, April 26, 2018, at the Multidisciplinary Living Donor Selection Conference. All elements of the medical and psychosocial evaluation including PHS increased risk were reviewed by Dr. Bentall, A. (3–4102). The patient was approved and the patient meets selection criteria based on age eighteen years or older, renal function, BMI, glucose and blood pressure within identified guidelines, including absence of significant co-morbid medical or psychiatric conditions and anatomy suitable for donor nephrectomy. Patient was approved and meets Mayo Clinic donor evaluation criteria. Patient was notified and verbalized understanding.

The following team members were present:

- Physician—agree with the recommendations

- Surgeon—agree with the recommendations
- Social Work—agree with the recommendations
- ILDA (Independent Living Donor Advocate)—agree with the recommendations
- Transplant Financial Services—agree with the recommendations
- Nutrition—agree with the recommendations
- Pharmacy—agree with the recommendations
- Living Donor RN Care Coordinator—agree with the recommendations

It gave me chills to see that long list of people. These eight consummate professionals, each at the top of their field, had gone on record to say they thought this was safe and reasonable for me to do. This was the referendum I had been waiting for.

Deb and I spent the next morning trading voice mails and text messages. She was going to a yoga class, and I was in a rideshare with Don on our way to the airport. He was going to Chicago for a national Jewish Family Services conference, and I was joining him for a much-needed mini vacation. I was still coughing, but I hoped that would soon taper off. One thing you learn pretty quickly in Transplant Land is that nothing is for sure for long. Now that I was approved to donate, Deb's team wanted to know whether we would consider a new option: Did we want to enter the Kidney Paired Donation program? It turned out that the possible issue with our blood crossmatch was real after all, one number that was higher than optimal out of all the numbers that mattered. It was not a big mismatch; in fact, it was small enough that Deb's transplant team had still "accepted" me as her organ donor. But her medical team thought there was a chance that she might do better in the paired program, possibly finding a donor with whom even that slight miss was missing. Would I be willing to try? Deb asked.

Of course we should try, I said.

Dr. Bentall had already brought up the possibility of the paired program and described the details. It seemed perfectly reasonable to see whether Deb could do even better by widening the pool. Furthermore, if we could help more people get the organs they needed through the paired program, then I was absolutely up for sharing the goodwill. Deb was too.

Deb asked whether I would mind that my kidney might not go directly to her. That did not seem important, I said. I would still be down a kidney. She would still be up a kidney. That was all that mattered. She felt the same.

The only downside seemed to be that the process would be more complicated, trying to schedule four, six, eight, or even more people for surgery, rather than just the two of us. But we both agreed that was a complexity we were willing to accept. And if we did not find a better match in the paired program, then we would proceed as planned with our directed donation. We would help more people if we could, but one way or another, Deb would get a kidney.

At the same time we were discussing the paired program, Deb and I were also finalizing a good backup surgery date in case that did not materialize. No matter what, our surgery had to be after Nathan's wedding on June 2. Don and I were also very close to making a deposit on a long-planned trip to Scandinavia in July. Should we hold off on making that financial commitment? Pay the deposit, Deb said. She wanted to spend the summer with friends and family in Florida before undergoing the transplant. She still had about 15 percent kidney function and felt pretty good. We would look for a date in the fall.

Lisa had explained that I needed to be at Mayo early in the morning the day before surgery for required pre-op tests. The nonhospital parts of the clinic were closed on the weekend, so that knocked out a Monday surgery date. There were also the Jewish

High Holidays to consider. At first, Don felt it was important for us to be in Kansas City to worship with our home congregation for Rosh Hashanah and Yom Kippur. Since Jewish holidays begin at sundown, our synagogue holds services over two days—evening and then morning. But as the list of available dates got pared down for other reasons, we both agreed this was definitely a case where *pikuach nefesh* applied. This is the principle in Jewish law that commands that the preservation of human life overrides all other religious duties. Finding a surgery date to donate my kidney was more important than going to services, even on the holiest days on the Jewish calendar.

Another major variable was surgeon availability. Deb was a complicated case, since she had already received both a kidney and a pancreas in her first transplant surgery. She had forged a relationship with Dr. Prieto, the transplant surgeon I had met during my March evaluation appointments, and she really wanted to select a week when he would be available to perform her surgery. We also had to pick a week when Mayo would have a transplant surgeon available for me, as well as two full surgical teams and two operating rooms.

After sifting through all the options and consulting with both our care teams, there was one standout date that met all the criteria— Tuesday, September 18. Deb's team was responsible for putting the surgery on the Mayo calendar; they booked it.

Our plan was set: If Mayo could identify a pair or chain for us before September 18, then we would go that route. If nothing materialized in time, we would revert to a directed donation, just Deb and me, on September 18.

We both loved that date: 9/18/18. In Jewish numerology, the number eighteen stands for "life." The next time the stars would be this aligned would be September 18, 2118—in a hundred years!

Even more propitious, this year Kol Nidre, the start of Yom Kippur, the holiest day of the Jewish year, would fall on the night of September 18.

I loved the idea that I was scheduled to share my spare kidney with Deb on the luckiest, holiest day in a century!

Of course, our first choice was still the paired kidney program. Not surprisingly, this meant a whole new set of requirements. Mayo needed my signed consent before they could start looking for a pair or chain match. The sooner I could get that back to them the sooner they could start searching. We got it done that day.

At this point, Lisa transferred my case over to Kay, the nurse transplant coordinator in Mayo's paired program. She would be the one to run daily searches against their database looking for a match. Dr. Bentall had explained to me that the Kidney Paired Donation program works with all the Mayo Clinics—which include their locations in Jacksonville, Florida, and Phoenix, Arizona, as well as "our" clinic in Rochester. That meant if the best recipient match for my kidney was a patient at Mayo Florida or Mayo Arizona, my organ might be removed in the operating room in Rochester and flown to one of the other locations for transplantation. In fact, the consent forms I signed acknowledged that I understood there was a possible risk of my kidney being damaged during transport. I hoped that was just a formality.

While we waited to see whether we would be part of another match, our regular lives moved on.

Don and I flew to Washington, DC, in May to spend Mother's Day with our daughter, Sarah, who had recently moved there for a new job. Sometime during that trip I stopped coughing—finally.

Nathan and Bridget had a beautiful wedding in early June. For the first time in half a year, thoughts of potential transplant surgery were far, far away, as we celebrated with my family, Don's family, our new in-law family, and Nathan and Bridget's friends. All my Omaha cousins and most of their spouses and children were able to join us in the Twin Cities. We did not talk much about my upcoming donation, but it was particularly special to be together with that branch of the family knowing what was on the horizon.

On June 7, just a week after the wedding, I got a text from Deb: "Call me please!!" Her nurse transplant coordinator had called to tell her they had identified six other people to "chain" with us—for an eight-person transplant surgery in late July! I called Lisa and Kay to see what else I could learn. There wasn't anything either of them could tell me. In an effort to protect the privacy of each person in the chain, the amount of information available to any one person was very limited. Kay called five days later—we were scheduled for chain transplant surgery on July 26. For the first time since this process started, it was Mayo pushing the schedule to get this done. Someone in our chain must need a kidney soon.

Kay said my "new" recipient was a patient at Mayo Florida. She was sending out another blood kit for me to return there to confirm the crossmatch.

Deb now thought it probably made sense for her to have surgery in Florida as well. Jacksonville was a five-hour drive from her home in Fort Lauderdale—much closer than Rochester. And it looked like her kidney was starting out there too. It did not make sense for both Deb and her kidney to fly to Minnesota.

I would still have my surgery in Rochester as planned. It was the easiest location for me, the only one not requiring an airplane trip. My kidney could be flown to Florida.

Deb and I would miss seeing each other after our surgeries. But we agreed we could talk and text and even Skype during our recoveries. It made sense for each of us to go to the Mayo Clinic closest to home.

I waited for my blood kit, but it did not arrive. I called Kay. Was this another shipping glitch? No, she said. She had canceled the blood kit. There was a problem with Deb's donor; they were calling off the chain. The only glitch was failing to notify me.

I was bummed. I had been enjoying the adrenaline high of the new mantra: we are going to save FOUR people. I called Deb. She was bummed too. This meant her "better" match was off the table, at least for now. And we had both canceled a lot of things to make the July 26 date possible on our calendars. Now all those appointments and meetings had to be rescheduled.

The costs, the hassles, and the barriers to donating just kept growing.

12

Complexities of Increasing Organ Supply

(JOHN)

The various matching and swapping arrangements previously described are difficult to implement. Transplantation is a procedure that is fraught with uncertainty. As Martha's story shows, it is difficult to schedule even one transplant in ways that are convenient for the donor and meet the needs of the recipient. The difficulties are multiplied when there are two or more transplants. What should happen if donor 1 gave an organ, expecting that the intended recipient would receive an organ from someone down the chain, and, for whatever reason, the chain fell apart? The chain could fall apart in all sorts of ways. A recipient could get sick. A donor could get sicker. The organ harvesting procedure could not go smoothly, and the first—or second—organ could be damaged. Or, if the donor and recipient are in different cities, there could be problems or delays in transport of the organ. The more complicated the exchange, the more likely things are to go wrong.

Today, there is an even more complex sort of arrangement that is being tried. An innovative program was recently initiated at the University of California, Los Angeles Medical Center that allows people to donate a kidney today in exchange for a voucher that a designated recipient can redeem for a kidney in the future if and when a kidney is needed. This approach was first developed when a potential donor wanted to give to a loved one who had a progressive kidney disease. The donor, however, was not young, and the loved one's disease had not progressed to the point where a transplant was needed. By the time that need arose, years in the future, the donor might be too old to donate; he might not even be alive. To solve that problem, the donor requested that, in return for donating to a stranger now, he would be given a voucher that his loved one could "cash in" at a future date to receive a kidney as part of a chain donation arrangement (Kritz 2017).

Each new and more complex elaboration of paired exchanges or vouchers increases the pool of people who can donate and increases the chances for people on transplant waiting lists to get an organ. That is a good thing. But these various arrangements also push the boundaries of our definitions of payment or reward for donation. They begin to look more and more like markets. And, in most countries, markets in organs are illegal. Of this, Mark J. Cherry, a professor in applied ethics at St. Edward's University in Austin, Texas, writes,

> The practice of issuing a voucher that can be traded in for a functional human kidney for transplantation at some point in the future is just one more step along the continuum toward a full-fledged market in human organs for transplantation. Much like cash, the voucher serves as a placeholder for something of value. Moreover, again much like cash, vouchers permit the interchange of objects of value (in this case kidneys) to be separated by time, even years or decades. . . . They look very much like a market in human kidneys for transplantation—albeit a heavily regulated and governmentally restricted barter market. (Cherry 2017, 510)

One can imagine ways of pushing the envelope even further. What if, instead of a kidney-for-kidney exchange, a person donated bone marrow and another donated a kidney? What if one donated time working for a certain charity and the other donated a kidney? What if one donated a kidney and the other gave money to the donor's favorite charity? At some point, it would seem simpler to just pay the donor for the kidney. Why not, as a matter of policy, take that step?

13

Going Public, Moving Forward

(MARTHA)

Deb and I decided it was time to go public on social media about our match.

A lot of people already knew, of course. Deb had informed her family, and I had talked to our children from the very beginning. I had also talked to a small circle of close friends—both in Kansas City and in other parts of the country. The day I got the official approval from Mayo, I had written an email to my extended Omaha family, letting them know what I was doing and how much I was thinking about Ann.

But I felt that Deb should get to take the lead in telling "the world" about our story. On the afternoon of June 21, she posted a long entry on Facebook, detailing the story of her first kidney-pancreas transplant nearly eighteen years ago and her more recent health struggles since the donated kidney began to fail. Then she shared our story:

> In March, I received a call from Mayo telling me that they had found a donor who matched. My guardian kidney angel. Martha Gershun a woman whose path I must have crossed a thousand times but whom I had never met, messaged me on FB to tell me that she was my donor and "just wanted to introduce herself."

What is the protocol for meeting the person who is saving your life? Do you invite them over? Take them to a fancy restaurant? Fly them to Hawaii? Being two Jewish women, we met for lunch. I cried. She laughed. But we never ran out of things to talk about. After we looked at our calendars for possible surgery dates (yes, we actually did that and settled on September 18th), we talked about our kids, her son's upcoming wedding, the cruise that she and her husband had planned for the summer, my youngest daughter's first year of college, how I liked being an empty nester now living on the beach in Fort Lauderdale.

When lunch was over (she let me pay, thank god) we hugged and I held on a little bit longer then I'd normally hold on to someone I had just met. She and I were bound together by something totally incomprehensible to most. None of us know how long we will live but, because of Martha's selfless act, I know that my immediate future looks brighter than it has in a while and I can make plans to live life again.

I posted a link to Deb's entry on my Facebook page:

Here is the other half of my "kidney story." Say hello to Deb, a beautiful, brave, delightful woman who just happens to need something that I have to spare. You can read more about her here.

The *Kansas City Jewish Chronicle* had published an update to Deb's story in mid-April under the heading "April Is Donate Life Month": "Gill tells us 'a wonderful woman reached out to be tested as a potential organ donor and was found to be a match. She is currently being evaluated for her general health, and assuming that they find no underlying health issues, we will be able to go ahead and schedule a transplant.'" The *Chronicle* went on to note, "Amazingly, the two women have crossed paths several times, belonged to the same congregation and organizations, but never met. We hope to provide another update soon."

This had launched quite a bit of quiet speculation in the Kansas City Jewish community about who had been identified as Deb's match. I was glad everyone now knew it was me.

People's reactions to the news were all over the map. Most either thought I was a living saint or a misguided fool. Many said they thought it was wonderful and expressed amazement that I had actually matched with a complete stranger. Those who knew my family story or who had known Ann and Cheryl in Omaha said they understood how meaningful this was for me. Those who knew Deb and her family thanked me profusely for stepping up to help someone they cared about. Some acquaintances shared their own family stories about kidney disease, organ donation, and other medical miracles. Some talked about the health problems that regrettably meant they could never donate.

But the most common sentiment I heard was "You're a better person than I am; I could never do that." This was typically accompanied with some version of the same concerns: What about the risks of surgery? What if your remaining kidney fails? What if someone in your close family needs a kidney in the future?

These comments came up so frequently that I developed stock responses: The surgery is very low risk. Almost no one dies during surgery to remove their kidney. While there is an increased risk of kidney failure with only one kidney, the absolute risk is still very low. The data shows kidney donors live just as long as everyone else. I trust Mayo's astoundingly rigorous evaluation process to be sure I am healthy enough for the procedure. I also explained that kidney donors are automatically registered with the United Network for Organ Sharing and receive preferential treatment if they ever need a kidney transplant themselves. People seemed to find that promise of a backstop reassuring.

As for the last question, I did not want people to think I was being cavalier about my family's potential needs. It was simply a matter of probabilities. Blood types are tricky, even among very close biological relatives, and my blood type, B positive, is one of the more restrictive. I could only donate to our daughter, Sarah, not to our son, Nathan, nor to Don. The very slim odds that Sarah, young and completely healthy, would need a kidney in the next ten years (assuming at some point I really would be too old to donate), seemed negligible. I could start a pair or chain arrangement to benefit one of my relatives, but again the rapidly diminishing useful life of my organs made this scenario highly improbable.

I asked our kids how they felt, since they were the people potentially most impacted by my decision. Sarah said she thought what I was doing was generous and good and she was proud of me. Nathan was equally clear: "I don't think our family should hoard kidneys."

It was hard to explain to people why it made me feel special to be able to do this. If there were no match criteria, if anyone who read about someone in need of a kidney could step up to donate, I do not know whether I would have. But because the odds had been so low, because I was now literally the only person in the world identified to do this for Deb, I felt chosen. Not in a God-pointed-a-finger kind of way; my own view of God did not involve that kind of individual, personal intervention. I felt chosen in a statistically-improbable-coincidence, mom-always-said-I-was-special kind of way. As unlikely as it was for any specific individual to match, I had matched. I had been given an astounding, improbable, winning-the-lottery chance to help someone else in this profound way.

Others thought I was special because I had agreed to do this; I felt special because I could.

People seemed more comfortable when they learned how our family experience with living kidney donation put this mitzvah on my radar. Since I had a close relative saved by a transplant, and they did not, that helped them absorb my decision to do something they did not want to consider for themselves. So I crafted an elevator version of that story and told it over and over: "My beloved cousin received a kidney from her dear friend in Omaha. I want to pay that forward." This was not my only motivation. Not by a long shot. But it was an explanation most people could accept. I was telling them news about my life, not suggesting what they should do with theirs.

14

The Countdown Begins

(MARTHA)

Once our chain fell apart, it was now most likely Deb and I would move forward with the directed donation on September 18. There was a chance that Mayo would identify another opportunity, but B positive is a relatively rare blood type so it was unlikely new matches would show up in the database in time.

Several weeks later, Don and I left on our much-anticipated vacation to Scandinavia.

We would have canceled the trip if it became necessary to make the transplant schedule work, but we were glad we did not have to. The trip was a magnificent reprieve from the stress of all the transplant machinations. When we returned in mid-July, I was refreshed and ready to confront the surgery in earnest. It became our top priority.

Don began conferring with Deb about hotel options in Rochester. We settled on a two-room suite with a kitchen at the Marriott Residence Inn right next to Mayo. Deb booked our accommodations.

I also set up a phone call with my friend Matt in North Carolina. Weeks earlier, Matt had posted to Facebook that he was going to be donating a kidney to his mother at Duke University Hospital. I was astounded at the news. Matt and I had worked together in Boston ten years before, when I was in the middle of my major effort to lose weight and get in shape. Matt was a long-distance runner who had trained people to run marathons. He offered to train me. I laughed him off: "I'm too old and too fat." He would have none of it: "I've trained people older and fatter than you."

For the next eight months, I religiously followed the training schedule Matt set for me, building enough strength and endurance to run my first Chicago Marathon in 2008. When I crossed the finish line, he was the first person I called. Now the coach who was responsible for my physical fitness, the person who literally made it possible for me to even consider donating a kidney, was donating a kidney himself.

Matt and I talked for nearly an hour. His surgery had gone well. There had been a brief blip when the surgeons found a cyst on his kidney, but a real-time biopsy done while he was still on the operating table showed it was "not concerning," and the transplant continued. Both Matt and his mother had recovered on schedule. He was now back at work as a marketing executive and had resumed his busy life as a community volunteer, husband, and father to two active, school-age kids.

Once again, Matt had good advice: bring a small firm pillow to Rochester so I could hold it against my abdomen to relieve pain at the incision site during recovery and the drive back home. He also encouraged me to be sure I had a supply of pain medication when I was discharged, regardless of my pain level while I was in the hospital. He had not done that, and he regretted it.

Other than the email a month earlier from the Kidney Paired Donation nurse transplant coordinator informing me that our chain had been called off, there was radio silence from Mayo. I found that both surprising and a little unsettling. The lack of communication made me feel like an inanimate input to their process, a stock part that everyone assumed would arrive in good condition on the appointed surgical date. But I was a human being with feelings, not inventory. I was anxious. I could have used a little encouragement.

It appeared Mayo's focus was on the beginning of the process, with their comprehensive evaluation, and the end of the process, with their excellent surgical and postoperative care. The middle was apparently up to me. Deb was not receiving any communication from her care team either, so we did our best to support each other, texting and talking on the phone from time to time. I was glad this was not an anonymous donation; I needed a partner to talk to.

As the surgery date loomed closer, I could not stand the official silence. I had a lot of questions about the exact details of my surgery and the recovery expectations, and I was having trouble making plans without the answers. I finally emailed Mayo to ask for details. And the frustrations continued. Lisa wrote back right away with some details about the surgery—that there would be lab work, that I would be in the hospital two days postoperatively, that I would have to take it easy for a month. Then she dropped a bomb. She said that the date of the surgery was not yet finalized. What?? Deb's care team had previously talked about it as a done deal. My anxiety started to spiral: We had hotel reservations. Don had made arrangements to be off work. We had plans! I called Lisa in a panic. She called back that afternoon and told me that yes, in fact, the date was set for September 18. I wondered if they were deliberately trying to drive me insane.

Then, when I looked over my notes, I noticed that federal law required HIV-hepatitis blood tests from all organ donors within twenty-eight days of surgery. I assumed I would be getting a kit on or about August 21 in anticipation of our September 18 surgery date. When August 21 came and went, I became anxious. The last time a kit had not arrived from Mayo, it was because they had canceled my surgery.

I emailed Lisa to ask what was going on. She wrote back, "I have not gotten the official notification of a surgery. I will however, order kits and let you know what I need you to do. I will order right away!"

Once again, I was shocked at Mayo's lack of attention to detail. Why did I have to trigger the order for a lab kit? I was turning my life upside down to volunteer for a surgical procedure to save one of their patients, earning them revenue and adding to their prestigious track record in the process. Didn't that make it their job to focus on the scheduling details, not mine?

I must have woken the system up, because I got another email from Lisa just minutes later, with template language saying they were required to recheck blood for HIV and hepatitis within twenty-eight days of all organ donation surgeries. I knew that; I had been the one to write to her.

The email said I should "Take this locally to have it drawn around the 4th of Sept and no later than the 10th of Sept." Now the real cost of Mayo's delay became obvious; that window was tighter than it looked. Mayo required the blood be drawn and shipped only on a Monday, Tuesday, or Wednesday, so it would arrive for processing before the lab closed for the weekend. That gave me only four possible days to get this done. Of those days, Monday, September 3, was Labor Day, when my doctor's office was closed, and Monday, September 10, was Rosh Hashanah, when I planned to spend the day at the synagogue. That left only two possible days for the blood draw, Tuesday, September 4, or Wednesday, September 5. I emailed Lisa and explained the kit had to arrive in four days for me to hit their window.

Lisa's email also detailed another requirement for this test: "It does require dry ice to mail it back. If your clinic doesn't have dry ice or charges for it, save the receipt and Mayo Clinic will reimburse you. If you need to locate dry ice in your community, try dryicedirectory.com."

The Dry Ice Saga

I did not know anything about shipping with dry ice. I called my doctor's office. They did not know anything about shipping with dry ice either.

I logged on to the website Mayo had suggested. Most of the listings near my zip code were grocery stores. I called several near my house. I learned that grocery stores only sell dry ice in ten-pound blocks, much more than I needed for this project. I wrote to Lisa for more suggestions. She had two recommendations: I could come up to Mayo—at my expense, of course—a few days before the surgery and get the testing done there. Or I could have them draw blood the morning of the surgery and "hope" they could run the test in time.

I was very annoyed. Mayo has been performing living kidney transplants for years—surely they could come up with a better answer to the dry ice problem!

I decided to try harder to solve the problem myself.

I had seen one local wholesale distributor on the Dry Ice Directory, listed in an industrial part of town that I did not recognize. An extremely helpful guy named Kevin said he would be happy to sell me a few pounds of dry ice. I should just call in advance the morning I wanted to pick it up to be sure the day's dry ice shipment had arrived. What if it doesn't arrive? I asked. I could hear him shrug over the phone. Hopefully that will not happen, he said.

I went to our local Hen House grocery to investigate backup plans. They sold dry ice, but they advised it would be dangerous to chop their ten-pound blocks into smaller bits. They did not have anyone on staff who would do that. They had a brochure for a product called "dry ice medical transport pellets." Ah-ha. That must be what Kevin was offering to sell.

I thought perhaps one of the larger national laboratory chains had a way to draw blood and ship it on dry ice. I could not get past the autoattendant that answered the phones for our local Quest lab, so I drove over to ask in person. They told me they did not have a partnership with Mayo, and they could not draw blood without a doctor's orders. Another dead end.

The dry ice warehouse was rapidly emerging as my best option.

But now I was not taking anything for granted. I decided to stop by the local FedEx store to confirm I could actually ship the stuff. Absolutely not, they said. The only FedEx depot in the region that could handle dry ice was the FedEx Shipping Center in Lenexa, twenty minutes away. "You know it's classified as a hazardous material by the Department of Transportation?" the guy behind the counter asked.

Actually, I knew no such thing. I was a prospective kidney donor, not a shipping expert. None of this was supposed to be my job.

I stopped at the UPS Store across the street to see whether I got a different answer. No; they would not handle a dry ice shipment either. I decided it would be wise to confirm my one and only shipping option and called the main FedEx 800 number. Yes, the main FedEx depot in Lenexa could accept my dry ice package as long as I used a government-approved shipping label. I was not sure what that meant, but I decided to worry about it later.

Now that I had a dry ice source and a shipping option identified, I called my doctor's office to be sure they could draw the blood on Tuesday. I was saving Wednesday as a backup. They could squeeze me in at 10:15 a.m.

It had taken me half a day driving around and making phone calls, but it looked like I had developed a dry ice solution that would work. I was very relieved.

I emailed the good news to Lisa and asked her to confirm the lab kit was on its way. She assured me that she had requested overnight delivery and it should arrive at our house the next day. I stayed home all day to wait for the FedEx delivery, but it never came. In the morning, I emailed Lisa in a panic; if the kit did not arrive by the next day, the Friday before the three-day Labor Day weekend, I would miss the 10:15 appointment on Tuesday morning to get my blood drawn. We would miss the window, a window made artificially short by Mayo's just-in-time planning process. It was known from the very start that this federally required blood test had to be done within twenty-eight days of our surgery date. Why not send out a kit much earlier and give living donors the luxury of time to arrange to get this done?

The kit will definitely arrive tomorrow, Lisa promised. We were cutting it pretty close, I thought. And now I would have to stay home another day to wait for the FedEx delivery.

I held my breath until the kit did, in fact, arrive midmorning the following day, Friday, August 31. The box included very intimidating instructions about how to label the return box so that the shipping company would accept it. This involved filling out the provided Class 9 hazard label (with very scary black stipes) and marking the box with the designation UN 1845, the net quantity of dry ice in the package in kilograms (side note, 1 kg = 2.2 lb.), and the name and address of both the shipper and recipient in durable ink. All this information had to be affixed directly to the package on the correct side. Also, I should be sure the box was sealed, but not completely or too tightly.

And those were the easy instructions; at least I could understand them. The instructions for the blood samples made no sense at all. I emailed Lisa again, who blithely wrote, "The lab will do this for you. Not to worry. It will be fine!" But I had already called my doctor's office, and they had told me they had no experience freezing specimens or shipping on dry ice. They could draw the blood, but that was it. I decided to call the lab at Mayo to try to get more useful information. The technician I spoke with told me the printed instructions were meaningless, and she had no idea why they sent them out. Mercifully, she said she would tell me exactly what to do.

It turned out not to be that complicated—though getting it wrong could have had serious consequences. I was to go to the distributor first and purchase enough dry ice pellets to fill the Styrofoam container, a ten-inch cube, about three-quarters full. Filling it to the top could be dangerous, the technician explained, because dry ice releases carbon dioxide gas which can build up enough pressure to rupture a package if it is packed too tightly; if you do not leave enough room, the box can literally explode in midair.

After I procured the dry ice pellets I was to drive immediately to my doctor's office for the blood draw. She wanted the office to spin the vials, then put them on top of the dry ice. According to the lab tech, they would immediately flash freeze.

Then I was to send the box back by FedEx.

I thanked the lab tech profusely. She was the first person I had talked to who actually seemed to understand how this HIV-hepatitis lab kit was supposed to work.

All Labor Day weekend, I fretted. What if something went wrong with the dry ice? What if something went wrong with the blood draw? What if I could not ship the kit back to Mayo on time? What if they had to postpone the surgery? I could not stop catastrophizing about the macro implications, too: if Mayo really needed more organs for their patients, and if living donors were a huge untapped resource, why couldn't they make it easier for us to do this very hard thing?

On Tuesday morning I got up early and called Kevin before seven. Yes, the dry ice shipment had arrived. I could come anytime. If the door was locked, he was just in the back warehouse; he would be back soon.

Kevin was happy to help fill my Styrofoam box three-quarters full with dry ice transport pellets. He had specialized gloves to handle the stuff, which hissed and steamed while he poured it in. There was a lot of paperwork he had to fill out, and I had to sign— most of it stating that if the dry ice harmed or killed anyone, Kevin was not liable. That was not reassuring. Then he warned me to keep the windows of my car open while I drove. Why? Because the carbon dioxide gas created by the melting dry ice can suffocate you in a closed space, he explained. Just recently he had a customer who died transporting dry ice in their car. That was not reassuring either.

I got in my car, rolled down the windows, and drove slowly, wind whistling through the open windows, to my doctor's office across town.

The blood draw did not go smoothly. The nurse said the written instructions did not match the vials in the kit, and she could not tell what they wanted. While she scrutinized the printed instructions, attempting to force them to reveal their secrets, I called the Mayo switchboard again. This time they were not as eager to put me through to the lab, but I begged and cajoled, and finally played my best card: "I'm a prospective living kidney donor. If you want me to do this, I need your help." That worked; I was connected to the lab.

Once again, the lab technician was extremely helpful. After getting instructions, the nurse drew my blood, carefully measured the correct amounts into four different vials, and spun them for the requisite time. Finally, finally, we labeled everything per Mayo's instructions, opened the steaming Styrofoam box, laid the vials on top of the dry ice, and quickly closed the whole thing before it could kill someone.

All my previous blood draws had taken five minutes, maximum. This entire process took forty-five minutes; when I left the office, there was a waiting room full of people whose appointments had backed up while the nurse helped me. I slunk out, feeling guilty, clutching my precious box.

I settled the cargo in the backseat of my car and headed to FedEx, where a very professional employee said they handled dry ice shipments all the time. I had done an excellent job with my labeling. He saw no issues; my package was on its way.

As all the built-up tension slowly subsided, I realized I was completely exhausted. I barely made it home before collapsing into bed alongside my cat, falling into a deep two-hour nap. The multiday ordeal acting as a shipping and phlebotomy expert had wiped me out. No matter how difficult the surgery turned out to be, I felt I had just completed the most difficult part of this mitzvah.

15

Ethics, Organ Markets, and Dry Ice

(JOHN)

Martha's dry ice saga graphically illustrates one of the central problems in organ donation today. We make it harder than it needs to be for people to donate organs. Advocates for markets in organs talk about the power of incentives. What we see, today, is the power of disincentives. It is as if transplant programs are willfully and counterproductively erecting barriers where they should be building on-ramps. There is no plausible reason why Mayo should not have had a system in place to help Martha ship her blood samples. If anything, the reason seems to be that hospitals are used to taking care of patients who are sick and who thus need the hospital's services and are therefore willing to put up with inconveniences and hardships.

But organ donors are not patients by the traditional definition. They do not come to the hospital because they have a health problem and need help. They are coming because they want to help someone else. They have much less incentive to put up with inconveniences and hardships.

Perhaps a better model is to treat organ donors the way we treat financial donors. Medical centers have excellent systems in place to deal with the altruistic people who want to make monetary donations. Philanthropy professionals in medical centers around the country are expert at taking care of donors, making it easy for them to give, cultivating them, and showing gratitude. Organ donation programs could improve their customer service, and possibly retain more potential donors, if they developed the ethos of their philanthropy departments instead of the ethos of their surgery departments.

Another sort of logic should also push us in the same direction— the logic of supply and demand. There is, today, a critical shortage of organ supply. The need to increase that supply should lead to efforts to remove, or at least reduce, the barriers of cost and inconvenience for people who are willing to donate.

There are lots of ways, both large and small, that medical centers could show gratitude and reduce barriers. They could treat organ donors and their caregivers to dinner or provide free hotel accommodations near the medical center. They could cover their out-of-pocket expenses. They could send thank-you notes. They could provide preferred free valet parking. They could make it easy to ship blood samples.

Such practices might look like the thin end of the wedge in a move toward paying for organs. But a fine distinction is important here. There may be marketlike innovations that would increase the supply of organs by helping potential donors overcome barriers and making them feel better about the process. That does not mean legalizing markets in organs.

Dominique Martin, associate professor in bioethics and professionalism in the School of Medicine at Deakin University in Victoria, Australia, and Gabriel M. Danovitch, the longtime medical director of the renowned Kidney and Pancreas Transplant Program at the David Geffen School of Medicine at University of California, Los Angeles, refer to this distinction when they write, "Advocates of financial incentive programs or 'regulated markets' in kidneys present the problem of the kidney shortage as one of insufficient public motivation to donate, arguing that incentives will increase the number of donors. Others believe the solutions lie—at least in part—in facilitating so-called 'altruistic donation'; harnessing the willingness of relatives and friends to donate by addressing the many barriers which serve as disincentives to living donation" (Martin and Danovitch 2017, 537–38).

Such innovations also push us to address a more fundamental question: What is wrong with legalized markets for organs? The idea of organ markets has passionate defenders and passionate detractors. Both rely on assumptions about what the effects of legalizing the sale of organs would be. Proponents argue that the current system is clearly inadequate. Too many people need kidneys, and too few people are donating them. As a result, patients on the waiting list are far more likely to die than they are to receive a deceased donor organ (Hippen 2005). If we could increase the supply of organs by creating a regulated market, we could increase the number of transplants and improve the health of people with kidney failure. This would also lower the cost of medical treatment for kidney disease since, in the long run, transplantation is cheaper than long-term dialysis (Jarl et al. 2018; Merion et al. 2005).

Opponents of markets paint a nightmare scenario of the poor being exploited as organ factories for the rich. They suggest the risks and long-term consequences are just too high to allow people to sell their organs. They decry an outcome whereby organ sellers will end up in worse health in order to improve the health of organ buyers. They argue this would increase health inequities and make those who are currently worse off even worse (Allard, Goldberg, and Fortin 2014).

One very odd thing about the debates about organ markets is that they portray the risks of donation as being very high. This is in stark contrast to the way that the risks are portrayed when they are discussed with unpaid donors such as Martha. Martha considered the risks, read reviews in medical journals, and discussed those risks with her doctors. All agreed that if she passed Mayo's rigorous evaluation, then the risks were low enough that donating did not seem likely to have a major effect on her life. Contrast that conclusion with the sorts of things that people write in describing the likely effect on someone who sells their kidney. Julian J. Koplin, a research fellow with the Biomedical Ethics Research Group, Murdoch Children's Research Institute and Melbourne Law School, the University of Melbourne, Australia, writes that kidney sellers "suffer adverse effects to their physical, psychological, social and financial well-being" (Koplin 2014, 8). He cites studies showing that vendors are at risk for renal impairment (Naqvi et al. 2008). Dominque Martin and Sarah White write, "[Kidney] vendors participating in regulated markets in developed countries would be at significant risk of adverse outcomes" (Martin and White 2014, 46–47). Other discussions of kidney markets use the same dire language.

There are some understandable reasons for this disparity in the forecast outcomes for organ donors. Where studies have been done of kidney sellers, they are in one of the very few countries where organ selling is legal, such as Iran or Pakistan. In those cultures, organ sellers tend to be impoverished, to not be screened well, and to not get good follow-up care. Their outcomes are likely more dire than the outcomes of voluntary donors in the United States, who tend to be well-off financially, be well screened, and receive excellent follow-up care.

But there is something else at work too. The outcome studies can be interpreted in different ways. Is a 1/2,500 risk of death after nephrectomy a "high," "moderate," or "low" risk? It is a number that can be categorized in different risk strata, depending upon the purpose of the categorizer. If the purpose is to encourage donation, it will be described as a low risk.

Also, the benefits to kidney sellers may be thought of differently than the benefits to voluntary donors. Donors receive intangible benefits. Sellers receive cash. Which is more valuable will depend upon the circumstances and the values of the person whose kidney is procured.

Defenders of markets insist that they can be well regulated and that the screening and follow-up for sellers would be the same as for donors. Thus, they argue, the outcomes would likely be similar to those for donors. Critics suggest that the existence of a cash benefit will encourage potential sellers to lie. If Martha, for example, had wanted to sell a kidney, she would have had a greater incentive to lie about her marijuana use. She might have chosen not to disclose her history of gestational diabetes.

The polarized debate about markets overlooks some features of the current system that could be fixed without necessarily legalizing markets in kidneys. Martha incurred significant out-of-pocket expenses in her efforts to donate, and she and her husband spent many days in pursuit of their transplant goal. She was fortunate that her recipient was able to reimburse her for their cash outlays and her husband had enough paid time off to allow him to serve as her caregiver. And Martha herself was retired from paid work, so she faced no lost wages by going through the donation process.

But that is not always the case. Fair compensation for those out-of-pocket expenses and time off work would not be the equivalent of a free market in kidneys. Rather, it would represent a reasonable effort to ensure no one has to lose money by donating a kidney.

We have no way of knowing how many potential living donors are dissuaded from donating because they cannot afford the process. But given the desperate need for more kidneys to help those on the waiting list, it would certainly make sense to remove these financial barriers to find out. Every new donor who is able to volunteer means a very sick patient might receive a lifesaving transplant, and everyone else moves up one slot on the transplant list. Why would we make people pay to participate? Why would we make people figure out where to buy dry ice?

16

Staying Healthy

(MARTHA)

With less than two weeks to go before the surgery date, I started to worry about getting sick. I knew that Mayo would postpone our surgery if I got so much as a cold, and I did not want to be the cause of any delays. I was going to avoid germs at all costs. Neurotically, I crafted a set of self-imposed restrictions. I would go out as little as possible. I would limit my participation in group gatherings. I would avoid shaking hands or hugging people.

That was easy enough to manage in my daily life, but it was going to pose a problem at our synagogue's upcoming Rosh Hashanah services, where hundreds of people would be gathering for worship, and hugging even casual acquaintances was the cultural norm. I decided to post on Facebook that I would be glad to see everyone, but I would not be hugging this year, and explained why. Most congregants were very respectful, and I managed to fend off the rest by taking a few steps back and offering a quick explanation. Even so, I found the evening Rosh Hashanah services very stressful, flinching whenever someone coughed or lunged to hug me without reading my body language. I decided to stay home from worship services the next morning, listening to Jewish music online instead of joining Don at Beth Torah.

For the past several months, I had been keeping to a rigorous workout schedule—at least sixty minutes of aerobic exercise every day, usually running and walking outside, but sometimes cycling on the stationary bike in our basement when the weather was bad. I had not skipped a day since we returned home from Scandinavia. I was determined to return to Mayo in the very best possible shape.

With eleven days to go, Mayo loaded my pre-op testing schedule to the portal. I had to laugh at the prep instructions. The day before surgery, I was to report to the lab at 6:40 a.m. for a urine collection. I was instructed to "please drink plenty of fluids" before arriving. The next test was a 7:00 a.m. blood draw. "Please do not eat or drink 10 hours prior to the test." I wondered if anyone ever thought to proofread these instructions; the conflicts were absurd. But I was tired of Mayo's inconsistencies. I had come to the conclusion that none of it really seemed to matter anyway or else they would have prioritized it.

With one week to go, I finished setting up the CaringBridge site that Don and I planned to use to keep our family and friends updated throughout my surgery and recovery. I sent out a large blast email so everyone we cared about would know this would be their best source for up-to-date information. Deb had set up a CaringBridge site too, and I provided a link for those that wanted to keep track of her journey as well.

Interesting packages began arriving at the house. My Omaha cousin Gail and her family in Denver sent a gorgeous soft blanket for my recovery. My Omaha cousin Donald and his wife Andi sent an actual greeting card that said, "Good Luck with your Kidney Transplant Surgery" (who knew they made things like this?). And my Boston sister Boo sent a book about two sisters and their bone marrow transplant journey, mostly because it had the words "sisters" and "transplant" in the blurb on the back.

My girlfriends were a tremendous support too. Kay, a recently retired school nurse, offered to drive to Rochester and stay with me overnight in the hospital so Don could get rest back at the hotel. I thought we had that covered, so she sent me off with a hospital care package instead. Gail, my weekly walking buddy, let me talk incessantly about all the preparation details so I could process everything that was happening while we traipsed the Kansas City streets together. Mary and Linda, fellow graduates of the Harvard Business School, shared my distress at Mayo's cavalier project planning, agreeing that this would all be fertile ground for numerous HBS cases.

Many more friends and family sent emails, messages on Caring-Bridge, and texts. One message, in particular, warmed my heart. A text from Ann's kidney donor, Cheryl, read, "Ron and I are in Italy—our first time ever! On our way to Florence from Venice via Verona today I thought of you! Please feel free to call me during any step of the way! Don, too. Ron and I are here and always part of the family. XOXO. Cheryl."

Don and I packed up the car to leave for Rochester. I was taking two bags—one for my time in the hotel, before and after surgery, and a smaller bag to take with me to the hospital. On Deb's recommendation, I had purchased a lightweight robe to cover my hospital-issued gown for post-op walks down the hall. I had also followed the suggestion of Judy, the lawyer who had donated a kidney to her mother, and purchased "grandma panties" that would fit loosely around my distended belly after surgery. They were not glamorous, but Judy assured me I would be glad to have them. I also packed my soft gift blanket, the firm pillow Matt recommended, Kay's care package, my knitting, two back issues of *People* magazine, a book by Philip Roth, and my laptop. I might be bedridden, but I had no intention of being bored.

17

First Attempt

(MARTHA)

We set out for Rochester at nine in the morning on Sunday, September 16. Don drove, while I texted with Deb. She and her boyfriend George were flying in from Fort Lauderdale early that evening. Cutting it that close would have made me incredibly nervous. What if the flight was delayed? Or, even worse, canceled? If it were me flying up to Mayo for life-saving surgery, I would have come days before, just in case. Deb and I had often joked that I was always early for things, while she was more of a "just in time" kind of gal. After the transplant, would she start getting places early too? We both doubted my kidney had that much power.

Deb posted a photo to her CaringBridge site from the plane, wearing a formidable face mask. Like me, she clearly was not taking any chances with germs. Deb and I were both anxious to get to Mayo and proceed with the organ transplant. Her health had been declining in recent weeks; she was exhausted and had been retaining a great deal of fluid. And I was growing weary of avoiding people and insects and infections. We had waited long enough; it was definitely time to get this show on the road.

As we got closer and closer to Rochester, I got more and more nervous. Up until now I had channeled all my emotional energy into the activities required to make the organ donation happen—pushing

Mayo to move through the process as quickly as possible, managing the evaluation and testing schedule, working to get my blood pressure down, handling the packing and shipping for the lab kits, and staying healthy. Now there were no activities to distract me; the only thing left was to show up at Mayo early the next morning to begin the final pre-op tests.

The enormity of this decision loomed. I was about to have major surgery I did not need with the accompanying post-op pain and a long recovery. I was going to let them take my fully functional, completely healthy, textbook-perfect kidney out of my body—and give it to someone else. I was going to let them put me to sleep whole—and wake up not. From the moment I learned I was Deb's match, I had wanted this. And I had gone to considerable effort to make it happen. I was relieved we had made it this far. But I was also scared.

Don and I did what we could to lighten the drive. We called the kids. They both wanted to talk and to hear how we were doing, but neither seemed overly concerned about the surgery. From the start, they had both been calm and practical about this project. If this is what their mother wanted to do, then they would be supportive. They were not overly dramatic, and they did not borrow trouble. I loved that about them.

Exactly halfway to Rochester, we stopped for lunch at the Gateway Market in Des Moines, Iowa, a surprisingly hip restaurant with delicious fresh and organic food. The menu was broad, with plenty of options for Don, who is vegan, and for me, a conventionally committed carnivore. Friends had recommended the place during our first drive up to Mayo. Since they were both restauranteurs and avid foodies, we took them up on the referral. We had such a good experience that "lunch in Des Moines" became a regular part of every drive to Minnesota.

The last time we had stopped there was on our trip home from Nathan and Bridget's wedding. I let those happy memories calm me now.

We arrived in Rochester in the late afternoon and checked into the Marriott Residence Inn for our long stay. We were amused at the placard on the small table in the kitchen–dining room listing resources to hire home health aides. I told Don I was glad I had brought him instead. Then we walked over to Charlton as a test run. As advertised, it only took a few minutes. We were set to go.

Pre-Op Tests

The morning tests were a snap after the rigorous three-day evaluation in March. Deb and George arrived just as I was returning to the waiting room after my 6:30 blood draw. It had been five weeks since our last visit in Kanas City, and I was distressed at Deb's condition. While she had mustered the energy to put on makeup and jewelry (more than I could manage this early in the morning), it was now abundantly clear that she was very sick. She had lost weight. Her legs and feet were puffy. For the first time since I met Deb, she looked like someone who needed a new kidney.

Don and I worked our way around the now-familiar Mayo campus, running through my pre-op appointment schedule like old hands. Lisa, my nurse transplant coordinator, was off that week, so the schedule directed me to Deb, also a nurse in the Transplant Center. I recognized her immediately as the teacher who had led our donor education class back in March. It was going to be complicated having a nurse with the same name as my recipient; other than that, I liked her a lot. She handed over two vital supplies— a bottle of powerful antibacterial wash that I was supposed to use in the shower that night and again the next morning and a prescription to take down to the hospital pharmacy for an equally powerful laxative which I was to take after dinner.

Nurse Deb took down my social security number and showed me the documents stating I was now registered with the United Network for Organ Sharing as a living kidney donor. It was official: if I ever needed a kidney transplant myself, I would receive extra priority "points" on the national organ waiting list.

Now was the time to ask the one question that had been on my mind for weeks. During the donor education class, Deb had mentioned that the two steps before surgery were putting in an IV and inserting a catheter. For reasons I can only attribute to my lifelong anxiety about finding a bathroom, I had fixated on the catheter, googling over and over to find out exactly how uncomfortable that was going to be. My girlfriend Gail had suggested a straightforward approach: "Just ask them to do it after you're under." But I was not at all sure I would be willing to be that assertive in the operating room.

I asked about the protocol. "We do that after you're under," Deb said, "Of course." And just like that, my very last obsession was dispelled. I dearly wished I had asked weeks before. But I probably needed something small and specific to focus on so I would not worry about the much bigger prospect of major surgery. Maybe the catheter was just the distraction I had chosen; if that had been addressed earlier, I suspect I would have quickly found something else to obsess about. And now, sitting in the consultation room with Deb, the nurse, it felt good to have something specific to be relieved about. Almost as if my psyche had planned it that way.

Dr. Prieto, the surgeon I had met in March, was going to perform Deb's procedure, so I had been assigned to Dr. Heimbach. I had looked her up before our trip and found her to be just as impressive as you would expect for a Mayo surgeon. She had been at the clinic since 2004. She was surgical director of Mayo's liver transplant program, with a special interest in improving outcomes for transplant recipients with obesity-related liver disease and striving to ensure long-term donor safety following living donor surgery. That sounded good to me. First, if her practice focused on operating on obese patients, I could stop feeling self-conscious about my less-than-flat belly. And second, I appreciated that my surgeon was focused on living donor outcomes.

I had also been secretly pleased when I learned I was being assigned to a female surgeon. It made my feminist heart happy. Now I appreciated the calm way Dr. Heimbach exuded competence and confidence. Plus, she got bonus points for very small hands. Kidney donor surgery is laparoscopic, except the single incision required for the surgeon to reach in and safely extract the kidney. My incision would be smaller thanks to Dr. Heimbach's petite hands.

Dr. Heimbach itemized all the risks of the surgery in agonizing detail, including the possibilities of bleeding and infection, and the unlikely event they would need to convert to an open procedure with a much more significant incision and longer recovery time. Then she had me sign numerous permission forms, saying I understood and accepted the risks. She asked whether I had any questions or concerns. I told her I had severe chronic dry eyes and that I needed eye drops several times an hour; I wanted to be sure that was noted for my care in the recovery unit. As soon as I was out of surgery, someone needed to be sure I had my eye drops. Other than that, I told her, I was good.

Next, the surgeon did a quick physical exam and confirmed she would be removing my left kidney. Then she took out a black permanent marker and wrote her initials on that side of my abdomen, "so everyone knows which kidney we plan to take."

I also had a final appointment scheduled with Margo, the social worker assigned to be my donor advocate. We talked about the upcoming procedure, and she asked what my plans were for after the surgery. I said I did not really have any. Margo immediately became hyperattentive. Had that question been more than small talk? Had I triggered a red flag that I might be suffering from depression? I quickly hastened to remedy any misimpression, explaining that it had been a very busy summer, with our son's wedding, our trip to Scandinavia, and numerous other projects, and I was looking forward to recovering without a long to-do list ahead of me. That was a gift I was giving myself. That must have done the trick, because she relaxed and asked a lot of questions about the wedding. She seemed satisfied that I did, indeed, have a great deal to live for.

Margo also asked if I wanted the Jewish chaplain to visit me in the hospital after my surgery. I declined, explaining the next night was Kol Nidre, the beginning of Yom Kippur, and I expected the rabbi would be very busy. I told her we were in touch with our rabbi at home and many friends from our synagogue in Kansas City, so I thought our spiritual needs were covered.

I had meant to save my complaints about the dry ice fiasco until after the operation. I did not want to be labeled a troublemaker before we even got to surgery. But Margo was such a sympathetic listener that I found myself telling her how frustrated I had been with the ridiculous effort to send my blood back to Mayo for the required HIV-hepatitis test. I was so keyed up that once I got started, I could not stop; I described in detail the extreme steps I took to get that done by the deadline and told her I really did not think it should be the donor's responsibility to handle things like that. What if donors lived in remote rural areas? I asked. What if they did not read English? What if they did not have the time or the skills to manage this project? What would that mean, I challenged her. With a critical shortage of organs nationwide, why would Mayo further reduce the pool of possible living donors by creating ridiculous hurdles like this?

I was pretty passionate, and Margo was taken aback. She said she had heard the dry ice shipping was sometimes an issue, but no one had ever described the problem in such detail. She was sympathetic and thanked me for sticking with the process. She would look into it, she promised. I did not have much confidence anything would change, but it felt good to have my say.

Don had a conference call for work that afternoon, so I made my own way to the EKG clinic, where I ran into Deb and George in the waiting room. He was now pushing her in a Mayo-issued wheelchair, where she was snuggled in the blanket I am pretty sure she had purloined from the first-class airplane cabin. Deb looked completely exhausted, though she was doing her best to stay cheerful. She told me they had decided to admit her to the hospital late that afternoon so they could run a full CT scan with contrast before our morning surgeries.

Deb was not excited at the prospect of one more invasive test and an additional night's stay in the hospital, but she was a trooper. She said she was glad that Mayo was being vigilant about her care. As always, I was impressed by her perseverance and stamina; the day was wearing me out, and both my kidneys were working just fine!

Throughout the day I was bolstered by emails, texts, and Caring-Bridge messages from friends around the country. My friend Jim called to wish me good luck from Kansas City. Many years before, Jim had a highly successful career in health care consulting, and he was my go-to friend for all things medical. His support meant a lot.

My last appointment was at 3:00 p.m. with Dr. Bentall. Once again the nephrologist would have the final say about whether we were approved to proceed.

I had a moment of panic an hour earlier, when my phone showed that one of the morning lab tests loaded up to the portal was posted in red with the flag "out of range." It was a positive result for cytomegalovirus. When I googled to learn more, the entry said it was harmless in most people but could be fatal to an organ recipient. Fortunately, Don had the good sense to look back at my earlier March labs; my test for cytomegalovirus was positive then too. Surely, he reassured me, they would have ruled me out back then if that was going to be an issue.

Dr. Bentall was smiling when he came into the exam room, charming as ever. I took the smile as a positive sign. He reviewed the lab results and consultations from the day's appointments. I asked about the cytomegalovirus result. He confirmed this was nothing to worry about. That reading is positive for more than 90 percent of adults in the United States; it just means sometime in my life I encountered that virus. He said they treat it like a blood type—some people are negative and some people are positive. They track it because they need to know which one I am, so they can adjust Deb's meds accordingly.

I told Dr. Bentall I thought "out of range" was a strange categorization considering those facts. He agreed, but said the doctors understood what it meant, and it was only an issue now that patients could look up their own results on their phones in the waiting room. I could not tell for sure, but I did not think he really approved of that innovation.

He also said my mini tirade (not his words) about the dry ice had gotten quite a lot of attention with the transplant team. I was surprised; it had only been a few hours since my conversation with Margo. How did they share information so quickly? Dr. Bentall told me they had heard complaints about the dry ice before, but my comments had been more "emphatic and articulate." I could tell he was amused. First the substance abuse appointment and now the dry ice protocol. I was getting a reputation.

Dr. Bentall said he was pleased that the replacement drug was working for my hypertension. He said the day's blood pressure readings were elevated, but that was to be expected before surgery. The earlier eighteen-hour home test was a much better indication that my blood pressure was under control. Then he cautioned that I would likely have to remain on the medication for good after the surgery.

"What if I follow your lifestyle recommendations and lose weight?" I asked.

"Consider that a challenge," he said. "If you do, then maybe we'll drop the medication."

Then the words we had been waiting months to hear:

"It's up to you," Dr. Bentall said. "We're good to go if you want to proceed."

Yes, yes, yes. I wanted to proceed. We were all good.

Don and I stopped at the pharmacy to pick up my laxative. Then we walked down the hall to scout out admissions; I wanted to know where I was supposed to report the next day.

All our errands completed, we walked back to the hotel in the late afternoon sunlight. I literally had nothing ahead of me but surgery. I told Don I was scared, that some part of me deep down wondered what I had gotten myself into.

"That makes sense," was all he said, and took my hand. He held it all the way back to the hotel.

The Speed Bump

I felt like I was in an altered state all evening. Every hour brought us inexorably closer to the surgery, and I did not know whether I wanted that time to go faster or slower. The odds of getting to this point were small beyond belief, yet here we were. I was going to donate a kidney to Deb.

I focused on staying calm as I moved through the evening's activities. I had been cautioned not to eat too much before surgery, and I did not want to go out, so Don and I ate a light dinner in our hotel room. I checked and rechecked my hospital bag. I drank the laxative, which tasted terrible. We settled in to watch the Emmy Awards while I caught up on last-minute email messages and well-wishes. I posted my carefully composed "Green light!" entry on CaringBridge and handed the site over to Don for a test message. I wanted to be sure he was prepared to notify our friends and family as soon as I got out of surgery. He reminded me that he was the technical one in our marriage, but I reminded him that I was the social media expert. I prevailed; under mild protest, he posted a test message.

At eight I called the Mayo automatic phone line to get my morning check-in time—5:30 for the 7:45 surgery slot. Assuming all went well, I would be out by eleven.

One last time, I made Don review the written list I had made for him to manage my postoperative care. I had kept it simple, and I had made him confirm it many times as we got closer to the surgery date: (1) Be sure I get my eye drops; (2) Be sure they give me as much pain medication as I need; (3) Post to CaringBridge so everyone knows I'm okay. And, of course, tell me how Deb's doing.

At eight thirty I took a shower, carefully scrubbing with the potent red antiseptic wash that was supposed to fend off any post-op infection. As instructed, I put on a clean nightgown and snuggled back into bed with Don to watch a few more Emmy Awards before we tried to sleep.

And then my phone rang. That telltale 507 area code. But I already had my surgery time; Mayo was not supposed to call tonight. I was very confused as I answered the phone. I did not recognize the name or the voice, a man with an unfamiliar accent who introduced himself as the transplant fellow on call.

"I'm sorry to have to tell you this," he said. "We're calling off the surgery tomorrow."

I couldn't move. I was sure it was a prank. All I could think was "This can't be happening. I've already taken the laxative."

Don told me later that I kept asking the same questions over and over, though it was clear that the doctor either did not know the answers or was not allowed to divulge confidential information about Deb's condition. What happened? Is Deb okay? Is the transplant canceled or just postponed? Am I supposed to pack up and go home? What am I supposed to do????

I was desperate not to let this unknown transplant doctor hang up. I had no way of calling back into Mayo that late at night and no emergency number to contact my care team in a situation like this. He was my only lifeline to Mayo, and I had to figure out what had happened and what it meant.

The doctor did not have many answers, but I gave him a lot of credit; he did not hang up. Technically, he was Deb's doctor, not mine. My doctors were all happily at home, oblivious that tomorrow's surgery was now called off. This transplant fellow did not have any responsibility for me, but he tried to help as best he could.

I finally got a vague picture of what was going on. Deb's doctors had seen something on the scans they had done late that afternoon, possibly signaling an infection in her lungs. If that was the case, it could prove very dangerous to start pumping her full of the immunosuppressant drugs required after a kidney transplant. The team had decided the safest course of action was to call off the surgery and wait until the infectious disease team could convene in the morning. Things might resolve in time to reschedule surgery in a week or so. He was not sure.

My situation had not been part of the conversation. All he could suggest was that I should call my nurse transplant coordinator in the morning. Perhaps they would know more then.

I finally let the poor doctor go and slumped down on the bed next to Don. He had gleaned enough from my end of the conversation to know that we would not be reporting for surgery in the morning.

"Should we start packing up?" I asked him. Which was a good indication that I was not processing very well. I had just swallowed a high-powered laxative designed to deliver a world-class cleanse. Obviously, we were not going anywhere right away.

"They'll need time to figure this out," Don said practically. "Maybe we'll go visit Nathan in Minneapolis while we wait. Let's get some sleep. We'll know a lot more in the morning."

But I was way too agitated to sleep. I did not think I should call Deb; I had no idea how she was feeling or how she was taking the news, or even if she was awake. But I wanted to make contact. So I texted: "Talked to the transplant fellow. I am so sorry! We will probably stay a day or two to see Nathan. I will come back WHENEVER you are ready!!!!!!!!!!!!!!!!"

She wrote back three words: "I love you."

I kept going over and over the new information, trying to reorient. There would be no surgery tomorrow. I had been given final approval, but there would be no surgery tomorrow. I had taken the laxative, but there would be no surgery tomorrow. Our family and friends were all thinking about me and sending up good wishes, but there would be no surgery tomorrow.

I felt like we needed to let people know, but Don and I both agreed I should not post to CaringBridge until we heard more from Deb. Our communities were closely linked, and if she had not yet told her family in Kansas City that the surgery was off, it was not our news to break. We had to give her time to communicate first.

But I wanted to talk. I called Gail. "You sound awful," she said. "What's happened?" I could barely tell her; it sounded like I was making it up. After everything we had gone through, it seemed impossible that the story had been derailed at the very last minute. After we hung up, I called Jim. For most of my life he had been telling me to be patient. Now he said it again. He was right. I should be patient. I would know a lot more in the morning. Then, still dazed and disoriented, I cuddled in next to Don and fell into a deep, dreamless sleep.

By two in the morning, the laxative had kicked in. After an urgent visit to the bathroom, I decided to check CaringBridge. Sure enough, Deb had posted.

Slight detour ahead
Journal entry by Deb Gill—Sep 18, 2018
There is no easy way to put this so I'm just going to say it. The transplant is being delayed until next week. It seems that I have a lung infection. The decision was made to NOT do the transplant this week but instead, to start dialysis tomorrow. I will receive 3 hours of dialysis tomorrow and every other day thereafter (Tuesday, Thursday, and Saturday) with the hope that the fluid and toxins in my blood stream are removed and the lung infection can be resolved so that the transplant can go forward next week.

My magnificent kidney sista, Martha Gershun, and her incredibly supportive hubby, Don, drove to Rochester yesterday and spent today running to lab draws and urine tests at 6:30 a.m., then to chest X-rays, EKG's, appointments with social workers, pharmacists, surgeons, nephrologists, etc. etc. etc. At 9:30 tonight, right after the doctor came in and talked to me, Martha received the news in her hotel room that the transplant was postponed. Her response? "I'll be here when you're ready." Who is this woman and where did she come from????????

Over this past year, I have often said that I feel like Wonder Woman when she is being attacked and using her bracelets to shield what is being thrown at her. (Notice I said "felt," not "look" like Wonder Woman.) It's been a visual that has helped me through some very rough times. Your messages have built me up and helped more than you know and I want to thank you from the bottom of my heart. I wish that I could answer every call and respond to each message but, Wonder Woman is just too beaten down and tired. I didn't know if or how I'd get through the disappointment tonight. Then I got Martha's message and it was the shot of adrenaline I needed. As with any good deed or charitable donation, in the end, she and Don get "nothing" tangible out of this benevolent act. They are doing it, she is doing it, because she is a good person.

Yes, I'm disappointed and yes, I am feeling sorry for myself. I even let myself cry tonight but, in the end, what good does that do? Martha is "there when I am ready." George is by my side. I am surrounded by family and friends and the best doctors in the world. My only job is to get ready, stay positive, get healthy, and do whatever it takes to see this through.

No one ever said that life is fair and even a superhero has moments in the movie when you're not sure she's going to make it. (But you know, deep down, she will because who would go see the sequel without her?) I too will get back up and fight this like I always have. I may just need a day or two to regroup and put my bracelets back on. 😴

Now I understood what had happened. I also saw that it seemed likely we would be proceeding with the surgery—just a week or two delayed. Since Deb had "gone public" with the news, I felt like it would be okay to tell our friends and family too. I went to the adjacent living room so I would not wake Don and, punctuated by trips to the bathroom, composed my own middle-of-the-night post.

Surgery postponed
Journal entry by Martha Gershun—Sep 18, 2018
We always knew there might be hiccups on this transplant journey, and last night we hit a speed bump (bad metaphor, I know). At 9:15 p.m., a few hours after I'd chugged down the requisite pre-op laxative and finished showering with the requisite pre-op anti-bacterial soap, I got a call from Mayo: The morning surgery was being postponed.

You can read Deb's full account here: https://www.caringbridge.org/visit/debgill.

I'm mightily disappointed, of course. We were so close! But the whole point—the only point—has always been to make Deb healthy. So if we have to go through a few more procedures, and if we have to wait a few more days, then that's what we're going to do. It will be worth it in the end!

I'll post updates as we learn more about our plans. Send your best prayers and healing thoughts to my Kidney Sister. She is fighting hard to get us back on our Transplant Track!

Then I went back to bed.

By eight the next morning I was able to get through to the Mayo Transplant Desk; they immediately put nurse Deb on the phone. She sounded just as shocked as we were. "I came in this morning and saw your procedure had been canceled. I've never seen them call off a surgery this close," she said. I asked her what the team needed me to do. Was I supposed to go home and wait? Stay in Rochester and wait? She did not have a lot of information, but said she would chase down Deb's care team and get back to me as soon as she could.

In the meantime, Don and I decided we would wait a few days before driving home. Up until the transplant was canceled, we had given very little thought to Yom Kippur. We just assumed we would be in the hospital for the holiday while I recovered from surgery. But now that plan was off, and we both agreed it would be too depressing to be on the road over Yom Kippur, the most somber day on the Jewish calendar. Plus, Don gets pretty spacy when he fasts for the holiday; a road trip did not seem prudent. We decided to stay in Minnesota and make the best of it.

I remembered that Margo, my donor advocate, had asked if I wanted to see the Jewish chaplain while I was in the hospital. Now I dug out Margo's business card and called to ask for help. Could she ask the chaplain to direct us to a synagogue in Rochester where we could worship for Yom Kippur? Margo was very sympathetic that the surgery was in limbo and eager to help. Less than ten minutes later she called back. The Jewish chaplain, Rabbi Michelle Werner, was also the congregational rabbi for B'nai Israel (Children of Israel), a Reform synagogue less than half a mile from our hotel "serving Rochester and worldwide visitors." Margo called the synagogue for us, and the staff said they would be more than happy to welcome us as guests for Yom Kippur. We would have somewhere to worship that night.

Meanwhile, Don called Nathan to confer about plans, given our changed circumstances. Nathan and Bridget had planned to attend services the next day at Shir Tikvah (Song of Hope), a Reform Jewish congregation in the Twin Cities with a mission of "radical hospitality." Unlike most synagogues in the United States, they did not require tickets or advance arrangements for the High Holidays; their services were open to all. Nathan suggested we meet at Shir Tikvah for services on Yom Kippur and then break fast together that night. There might even be time between morning and afternoon services to stop by their apartment and play with their dog.

I was still pretty dazed by the sudden turn of events, but it helped to have our plans for Yom Kippur in place, and I was very glad we would get to see the kids.

Deb texted: She had a "hall pass" to get out of the hospital for an hour. She and George planned to walk to Pannekoeken, the famous Dutch pancake restaurant around the corner, to have brunch with her mom and brother, who had arrived yesterday to be in town for the surgery, and would now be driving back to Kansas City. Did we want to join them?

Don and I walked over to the restaurant, where we all sat around a large round table for a veritable feast. For all the fast conversation and easy laughter, no one would ever guess the group was reeling from some very disappointing news. This was our most serious setback yet, but Deb was determined to stay positive. Her ironclad optimism was inspiring. We were determined to hang in there too.

Deb had talked to a wide array of medical professionals that morning, so she had more information to share. The infectious disease specialist was running lots of tests, but he thought the problematic shadows on the lung scans were due to fluid buildup and not an infection. That would be a much better scenario. We would know more in three days, when the full test results were in.

Meanwhile, Deb's nephrologist decided to postpone dialysis to see whether heavy doses of IV diuretics would take care of the fluid buildup. It had only been a few hours, but so far, that approach appeared to be working; Deb had already shed several pounds of liquid. The team was hopeful that once the excess fluid was decreased, they would be able to see her lungs more clearly. If there was no infection, and if everything else looked good, we could reschedule the transplant.

I talked to nurse Deb again by phone, and she told me it now looked like we would be back on the surgery schedule for the following week. She assured me that most of the tests and appointments I had done the day before would still "count," as well as the HIV-hepatitis tests that had been sent up on dry ice; other than fresh lab work and another nephrology appointment the day before the new surgery date, I would remain "cleared to go."

Given this information, Don and I settled on a plan: we would attend Yom Kippur Kol Nidre services that night in Rochester and then drive to the Twin Cities the next morning to spend Yom Kippur day with Nathan and Bridget. We would break the fast with the kids, drive back to Rochester for the night, and then drive home to Kansas City on Thursday morning, where we would wait to hear when we should come back for the transplant.

That afternoon I got an email from my Omaha cousin Donald. He reminded me that Ann and Cheryl's transplant hit a similar bump in the road. The night before their scheduled transplant, the hospital called to say they were no longer a match and everything was canceled. Ann and Donald's two adult daughters had traveled to Omaha, and the entire family was gathered for the surgery; everyone was devastated. But Cheryl refused to accept the doctors' pronouncement, and another series of tests proved she and Ann were compatible. Everything was postponed for two months, but the transplant eventually happened, and, of course, Ann lived for many more years. I was grateful to Donald for reminding me of that part of the family story. Ann eventually got her transplant; I believed Deb would too.

The night I was supposed to be recovering from surgery, Don and I instead walked to B'nai Israel Synagogue for a warm and meaningful Kol Nidre service. This lovely small congregation has a mission to welcome and comfort their many guests undergoing procedures at Mayo and their caregivers. Their *misheberach* (healing) prayer was the most beautiful I had ever experienced. The rabbi gave a lyrical, poetry-filled sermon on the spirituality of Torah. And she exhorted everyone to "choose life." Which was, after all, why Don and I were there.

The next morning, we drove ninety minutes to the Twin Cities for services at Shir Tikvah. As we were settling into our seats in the vast auditorium they rented for Yom Kippur, I got a call from 507. I slipped out to talk. It was nurse Deb. They had tentatively rescheduled the surgery for the following Wednesday morning. Deb's care team would convene on Monday afternoon, review all the test results, and make the go / no go decision. If the answer was positive, I would need to be at Mayo early Tuesday morning for pre-op labs.

Wait, I said. Do you expect us to drive all night to get to Mayo?

What do you mean? nurse Deb asked.

I will be coming from Kansas City, I reminded her. If you call me on Monday afternoon to say the surgery is back on, and you need me in Rochester by Tuesday morning for pre-op labs, then we will have to drive through the night to get there. That does not sound like a very good plan.

Oh, she said, sounding confused. You don't live nearby? I did not say anything, but my thoughts were not kind. Surely they could keep track of where their organ donor lived. It was another reminder of my peculiar role in this process—part patient and part supplier. Mayo had systems for each, but they did not have good systems for someone who was both.

Can you waive the pre-op labs the day before? I asked. No, nurse Deb was adamant. The pre-op labs were nonnegotiable. Then Wednesday surgery won't work, I said, equally firm. We are not going to drive through the night to get to Mayo. If Deb's team was going to make their decision on Monday afternoon, then the earliest I could be on the road was Tuesday morning. That meant the soonest I could present for early-morning lab work would be Wednesday. The math was easy: we needed a Thursday surgery date.

Nurse Deb put me on hold while she scrambled to find Deb's care team. She returned to the call. They could not get a surgical team together for Thursday, but they could do it on Friday. Dr. Heimbach would be out of town, but Dr. Prieto could do my surgery. But I thought he was Deb's surgeon, I said. He will do both procedures, the nurse explained. He can finish your surgery and then go into the next room to do hers.

The delay must have magically empowered me, because I held firm a second time that day. No, that is not okay, I said. From the start everyone has explained that my care team is focused on my best interests. If Dr. Prieto is Deb's surgeon, then how can I rely on him to stop midsurgery if I am at risk, when he knows she is in the next room waiting for my kidney? I did not get an answer to my question. But nurse Deb told me they would find a different surgeon.

I slipped back into the auditorium just as the liturgical music was beginning. "I think it's going to be Friday," I whispered to Don. And then we were immersed in the somber, introspective worship of Yom Kippur, the Jewish Day of Atonement.

Don and I broke the fast with Nathan and Bridget at a favorite diner near their home, and then set out to return to Rochester. It was a cloud-covered, rainy night, and the long drive through rural Minnesota was dark and dreary. We talked about the revised schedule and how we were going to reorganize our lives to make it work.

I would have to cancel my trip to Boston for my Harvard College and Business School reunions. The timing had always been tight; this delay almost certainly meant I would no longer be recovered enough from surgery to travel for the reunion festivities. I was sorry to miss both events, especially my college reunion, which I had been helping to plan throughout the summer. But the transplant took priority. My friends would miss me, but they would understand.

The reschedule was also going to play havoc with Don's work responsibilities. Not only had he missed three days of work for this first aborted surgery, but he was now going to have to miss an additional six days for the second attempt, with very little time in the office to catch up in between. That is a lot of time off for the CEO of a midsize human services agency, and Don was worried about the meetings he would miss and the added stress this would put on his staff.

It was ironic that after all our efforts to pick a surgery date that would work for Deb and work for me and work for Don, none of that careful planning mattered now. Our determination to pick an optimally convenient transplant date meant nothing in the face of the medical realities. The new surgery date might be inconvenient for me and terribly inconvenient for Don, but our scheduling issues had become irrelevant. All that mattered now was getting Deb her kidney.

The next morning we checked out of the Marriott Residence Inn and rebooked for the following week. They did not seem at all surprised. Apparently, it is common practice for Mayo patients to change their travel plans with little notice.

And then we drove back home.

The partial week back in Kanas City was surreal. I still did not want to be around crowds or people with germs, and I did not want to be too available to the mosquitos or oak mites that were lingering from summer. Friends had lined up to bring me food and keep me company while I was recovering from surgery—but now all those visits had to be postponed. I had nothing on the calendar and no purpose other than to stay healthy while I waited to hear from Mayo. I was a vessel, carrying a kidney.

Deb and I texted back and forth. She had been released from the hospital but had to stick close to the clinic, where she reported every morning for labs and every afternoon for a consultation with the nephrologist. Things were looking good, but we would not know anything for sure until her final comprehensive evaluation on Monday.

On Monday afternoon, I was having chia seed pudding with Kay at our favorite restaurant, trying not to keep looking at my phone. Deb had posted a photo to CaringBridge: She was at Mayo, on the exam table, she wrote, "trying to keep my sense of humor," while waiting for the nephrologist to bring the news. Deb was clearly holding her breath; I was too. It seemed like this entire year I had been waiting for phone calls from 507.

My phone finally buzzed; it was nurse Deb. The surgery was back on!

Please arrive at Mayo on Thursday morning for pre-op labs. You are good to go for Friday morning.

I exhaled. Kay and I high fived. I texted Deb to confirm she had heard the same thing. Yes, her team also said we were good to go. I texted Don to tell him we were back on.

The next day I passed the time visiting with girlfriends and went to my favorite spa for a high-end pedicure. Then I went home to wash and iron clothes, and we repacked to return to Mayo.

18

Second Attempt

(MARTHA)

Fall had begun to descend during our brief time at home, and the leaves were visibly turning as we passed through Missouri, Nebraska, Iowa, and finally Minnesota. This time, the drive was significantly more relaxed. There was nothing more to worry about. We just had to get to Mayo and repeat.

Six days after we had checked out of the Marriott Residence Inn, we checked back in. Deb and I had texted about possibly meeting up for dinner, but our timing was slightly off. I had to begin fasting early in the evening for the pre-op lab work the next morning, and she had just walked into a salon to get a mani-pedi. That made me laugh; we were both clearly determined to have well-done nails prior to surgery.

That night, PBS was rebroadcasting their two-hour Ken Burns documentary on the Mayo Clinic, so Don and I settled in to watch. We were particularly interested to learn how Mayo had developed their integrated approach to diagnosis and care, which included creating their own medical records system long before programs were commercially available. We also learned that Mayo physicians were all on salary, and not compensated per procedure, which is the norm in most hospitals. The documentary suggested this meant Mayo doctors were more willing to spend time with their patients, a practice we had definitely noticed. This was the kind of TV show that made you think, "If I ever need first-rate medical attention, I'm going to Mayo." And here we were.

The next morning, we met up with Deb and George in the waiting room of the Charlton lab. Deb was tired, but she looked good. More than a week of treatment had successfully drained most of the excess fluid she had been retaining. The powerful diuretics had done their job. But the same drugs can also damage the kidneys, especially when they are already weakened. Deb's kidney function was now down to virtually zero, making the transplant more critical than ever. We both hoped the day's appointments would be perfunctory and we would be approved for surgery the following day. Deb's life depended on it.

Lisa, my nurse transplant coordinator, was now back in town, so she took over from nurse Deb. I was very glad to see her again. She told me that the whole transplant team had heard from Margo, my donor advocate, about my dry ice story. She said the nurses had been complaining about this process for some time, but had not gotten much traction; she was not sure, but she thought my "passionate and articulate" description of the problem might help motivate change. Then she handed over my second bottle of antibacterial rinse and the prescription for another bottle of laxative. I knew the drill.

Since Dr. Heimbach was out of town, and I had declined to be operated on by Dr. Prieto, who was Deb's surgeon, I had been reassigned to Dr. Taner. I looked him up online and was once again impressed with this Mayo surgeon's extraordinary credentials.

In person, Dr. Taner was just what I had come to expect—quiet, competent, kind, and good-looking. It was like they were hiring out of central casting.

Dr. Taner apologized that regulations required him to read me the entire list of surgical risks again and obtain a new signature on the consent forms. Then he examined my belly and confirmed he would be removing my left kidney. He wrote his own initials on the left side of my abdomen where Dr. Heimbach's initials were now fading. Then he handed me the pen with a flourish. "You might as well keep it," he said. "We aren't allowed to reuse them."

I hopped off the examining table; we were almost done.

Dr. Bentall was unavailable that day, so my final "sign-off" appointment was with a different nephrologist, Dr. Taler. As before, the nephrologist's approval would be required for us to proceed to surgery the next morning. I assumed this appointment would be a slam dunk, since I had been approved the week before by Dr. Bentall, but there was nothing pro forma about Dr. Taler's exam. She slowly reviewed all the previous information and then looked very closely at the day's test results. "Your blood pressure is high," she said. I acknowledged it was always high when I was at Mayo, but explained that Dr. Bentall had felt the eighteen-hour results were a better indication that the medicine was keeping everything under control. She scowled. Oh my God, I thought. Is this last doctor at this last appointment on the very last day of this entire process going to say no?

But she just nodded. "I have to do my own due diligence before I can sign off," she said. "If you agree to stay on the blood pressure medication after the surgery, then you're approved." Of course. That had always been the plan. I quickly agreed, before she could change her mind.

At 4:38 p.m., I texted Deb: "Just finished with the nephrologist. We are approved!!! Sleep well. See ya tomorrow." I finished with a couple of kiss-blowing smiley-face emojis.

Don and I began a repeat of our pre-op evening ritual in the
hotel. This time was much easier. I was no longer scared; I just
wanted to get it done. At Lisa's recommendation, I had moved
to an all-liquid diet in preparation for the surgery, and Don
heated up several different kinds of low-sodium soup. Then
the shower with the antibacterial soap. Then the laxative. Then
I called the Mayo phone line. Since the hospital did not typically do transplant surgeries on Friday, I knew we would be first
up. Sure enough, I had a 5:30 a.m. call time for the 7:45 a.m.
surgery slot.

Last time Don and I had watched the Emmy Awards the night
before my scheduled surgery. This time we watched the Senate
confirmation hearings for Brett Kavanaugh's appointment to the
Supreme Court. I was not sure this was good for my blood pressure, but it kept me distracted. I posted to CaringBridge: "The docs
say we're good to go! Don will be the 'keeper' of this CaringBridge
site for a while; be kind to him. See you on the other side. Second
time's the charm!"

When nine and then nine fifteen came and went without a
phone call from 507, I began to fully relax. It looked like this time
would be a go.

I did not sleep much that night, as the laxative did its job again.
We finally got up around four thirty, and I showered once more
with the special antibacterial soap. It was too early for our check-in
time, but Don agreed we could walk over to Mayo anyway. I was
very nervous, and I knew I would feel better once I was at the hospital and proceeding with the day's activities.

I had anticipated a long queue at the check-in station, along
the lines of the Charlton lab, but there was only one other couple
ahead of us. Mayo must be used to anxious early arrivals, because
one of the receptionists opened up her station before their posted

hours and checked in the first patient and then me in under five minutes. The entire process was simple—no forms, just present your ID, sign the computer screen, and you are on your way to the next admitting station.

We were ushered to a private room, where I got to don a substantial paper gown that was so complicated they actually had instructions posted to the wall showing how to put it on. The admitting nurse asked every imaginable question, typing results into Mayo's computer system, and then they wheeled in a portable standing scale to weigh me. That was pretty clever. No wandering around the halls in that revealing gown. Then, best of all, the admitting nurse connected a wide, flexible tube from the wall to a port in my gown—and showed me how to adjust it to get hot or warm air—whatever I wanted.

I explained again about my serious dry eye condition. I wanted to be sure I could have easy access to my eye drops in recovery. The nurse took my bottle, the one I kept with me at all times, and gave it a bar code with my name and patient ID number, scanned that info into the electronic medical record system, then handed it back. "We'll take the bottle right before we put you under," she said. "We'll put it with your glasses, and you can have it back when you wake up." That sounded reassuring. Nothing panics me like being without my eye drops.

Now we just had to wait. No one was hovering, but I also felt like we were never far from help if we asked. That pattern would repeat often over the next few days.

When one of the nurses checked in, I mentioned that I was feeling slightly nauseous from the overnight laxative. "We have something for that," she said. I was expecting a pill or a shot—something high-tech and scientific—but she returned with a small plastic packet adorned with the Mayo logo containing a sample

size of eucalyptus. She instructed me to inhale from the bag periodically and let her know if that helped. It did.

Then it was time to unplug from the warm air system, say good-
bye to my husband, and go upstairs to pre-op. A nurse provided
detailed instructions so Don could track my progress during surgery. The team would text updates to his cell phone. Every patient
was also given a unique number, and they would post updates to
a "tracking board" in the transplant surgery waiting room. If Don
watched my number, he would know where I was at all times. That
suited my high-tech husband. And I was happy to be kept track of,
even if it made me feel a little like an airplane being monitored by
air traffic control.

Pre-op was a very busy place, a large room with twenty or more
hospital beds and lots of staff bustling around. It was also cold
and sterile—you could tell things were starting to get serious.
I climbed up on my designated bed and was immediately surrounded by techs, nurses, and doctors, each with a specific role.
The best part was the warm blankets they magically produced
from a warming cabinet to guard against the chilly room. The
anesthesiologist came over to introduce himself and confirm lots
of information. He explained that they would give me a kind
of spinal block at the very end of the surgery so I would wake
up with very little pain. Then he put a small scopolamine patch
behind my ear to control nausea after the surgery. It seemed they
thought of everything.

Then Deb arrived! We had thought we might meet up at check-
in, but true to form, I had been early and she had been late. We
joked again: Would that change when she got my kidney?

They gave Deb the bed next to mine, so we could talk while
everyone bustled around us. We were both pretty upbeat, very
excited this was finally happening, and we shared "our story" with

anyone who would listen: we had been strangers before I read about Deb in the newspaper; I got tested, and we learned we were a match; we had to postpone the first transplant; now, today, she would finally get my kidney.

I would go first; Deb would follow in about an hour.

When they came to wheel me into surgery, we gave each other an enthusiastic thumbs-up. Deb's big smile was the last thing I saw as I was rolled out of the room.

The operating room was small, cold, brightly lit, and filled with high-tech gear. I did not understand why they do not knock you out before you get there, because there is absolutely nothing comforting about that scene. I was asked to climb from my bed onto the operating table, fitting my body into a hard foam cradle. Now things moved quickly. Techs on either side put my arms on table extensions and prepared to insert IV lines. The tech on my left side was aggressive and clumsy with the tourniquet which pinched my skin. For the first time in my entire Mayo experience, I yelped: "That hurts." He was unsympathetic. "You'll be out soon," he responded. Which was true. After that, I was out.

Successful Surgery

The surgery went well. Don kept our friends and family informed on CaringBridge:

Martha is on her way!
Journal entry by Don Goldman—Sep 28, 2018
According to Mayo's high-tech (and of course HIPAA-compliant) system, Martha is in surgery. I can tell this both because her (secret) ID has turned orange on the Board and because I got a text. I wonder when they'll link their system to Facebook and Twitter. Thanks to all our friends, family and co-workers for all your support!

And then . . .

> Martha's done! I just talked to the surgeon. Martha's surgery is
> complete. She is doing well and I'll see her after she's out of recov-
> ery in a couple of hours. I'll keep you posted as her recovery pro-
> gresses. Next stop for her kidney, Deb Gill!

I woke up in fits and starts, fixating on the red, patterned scrub
cap which came in and out of focus above me. It belonged to the
nurse who appeared to be assigned full-time to my bedside. I do
not think she left me the entire time I was in recovery. As promised, as soon as I could open my eyes, the nurse put eye drops
in for me, then handed me the bottle so I could manage subsequent applications myself. When I finally woke up enough to talk,
I asked the same question I always ask coming out of anesthesia:
"What time is it?" About eleven o'clock. I felt no nausea. I felt no
pain. I could not feel the catheter. I really could not feel much of
anything, except my left arm, which was sore where the tech had
left a blossoming bruise when he carelessly tied the rubber band
for the IV. Other than that, the Mayo pain regimen was clearly
working.

By the time I could suck on ice chips, I was ready to leave recovery. In all the hustle and bustle of getting settled in my hospital
room, I could not see Don. I panicked. But then he was there, with
my extra bottle of eye drops, looking attentive but not at all worried. He had already called our kids to tell them I was fine. He told
me George reported that Deb was out of surgery and in recovery.

Best of all, George told Don to tell me that the transplanted kidney was making urine! Exactly nine months to the day after I first
read about Deb in the *Kansas City Jewish Chronicle*, my left kidney
had been surgically removed and successfully transplanted, and
now it belonged to her. It had taken as long as it takes to make a

baby, but we stuck with it—Deb and George, Don and me. And we did it. I felt sleepy, but very triumphant!

Rapid Recovery

The next two days in the hospital were a blur of activity and progress. I was allowed to eat immediately, and I was really hungry. We phoned lunch orders from the robust Mayo "room service" menu. Because of HIPAA, no one on staff could provide us with an update on Deb. We would be reliant on George for information, and he was still in the waiting room while Deb was in recovery.

I had heard horror stories about hospital staff being unavailable when patients needed pain relief, and had experienced similar issues getting my mother's needs met during a hospital stay in Kansas City decades before. So I had obsessively reminded Don to be hypervigilant on my behalf. But I was in very little pain, and nurses were constantly stopping by my room to check in.

Equally reassuring, the physical layout of the surgical floor was designed to give patients immediate access to help if needed. Each wing was an elongated oval, with rooms along the perimeter, and the well-staffed nurses' station in the middle. No room was more than twenty feet from multiple nurses at all times. Don could have walked out of my room, and he would have bumped into a nurse; I could have yelled, and someone would have heard me. The entire environment was comforting and safe. I had everything I needed, and it turned out I did not need very much.

Sometime after lunch, an older couple I did not recognize appeared at the door to my room. The gentleman introduced himself as a retired transplant surgeon who worked for many years at Mayo. The couple were family friends of Deb's sister. They had come to visit Deb and wanted to meet me. They were very gracious. Meeting someone who had been involved in this work from the very early days of transplantation made me feel part of something very big, as well as something very particular.

George stopped by. He explained that Deb had stayed in recovery longer than expected, while they gave her blood and started pumping her full of massive amounts of immunosuppressants to keep her body from rejecting the new kidney. But she was now up on the surgical ward, in the wing opposite mine, and doing well. I could go visit as soon as I could walk that far.

By midafternoon, a nurse came to see whether I could get up and move. I was very tentative about testing my stomach muscles. It was hard to sit up, but the transition from sitting to standing was not bad at all. One lap around the nurses' station was enough, though.

I had always assumed Don would spend the first night in the hospital with me, but I was doing so well we agreed it would be fine for him to go back to the hotel to sleep in a real bed. I slept heavily, waking up only when the nurse came in to take my vitals or administer my every-four-hour pain medication. Sometime around six in the morning (it was still dark), she woke me to say it was time to get untethered. She quickly removed both IVs and the catheter; I was free.

Don arrived an hour later, and we settled in to see what the day would hold. By midafternoon, I was ready to post to CaringBridge.

Day 2
Journal entry by Martha Gershun—Sep 29, 2018
As forewarned, the surgical spinal block wore off overnight, so I'm feeling some discomfort today. But this Mayo team is great at pain management, and so far I haven't needed more than the first line meds.

Don ordered me scrambled eggs and half a bagel.

The surgical and the medical teams think I'm doing great. They unhooked all the tubes and bags this morning, so I'm free to move about as I choose, though I tire almost immediately.

My main challenge for today is to pee, now that the catheter has been removed. Those who know me well will appreciate the irony.

Deb is in another wing on this floor, and my next project is to take a very slow walk in that direction. Deb's sister reports via text that Deb will soon be walking, too. So, hopefully, we can meet half way.

After several laps around the nurses' station, punctuated by periods of rest and intermittent cat naps, I decided it was time to walk over to Deb's wing. Don helped me make the slow trek down the hall. Seeing her lying in bed with a big grin, I felt the most tremendous relief and gratitude. And there, at the end of the hospital bed, was a clear bag filling with light golden urine—my kidney, her kidney, was working!

We swapped recovery stories and jokes, nothing sappy or maudlin. We were definitely alike that way.

Deb's surgeon had shared a story she was eager to share with me. Apparently, something happened while they were removing my kidney, and the renal vein was damaged. Deb was not clear on the details—whether it had been cut too close or damaged during the cauterization to control my bleeding, but in any event, the part that would normally be used to connect to her body had been damaged. Fortunately, she had enough remaining vein in her body that they were able to use that for the graft instead, and everything was fine in the end. I had not heard the story from my surgeon during rounds that morning, and no one else mentioned it while I was in the hospital. I thought perhaps HIPAA mandated that was information that should be disclosed to Deb (after all, once it was severed from my body, it was her kidney) and not to me—since it had no impact on my health or well-being. I never found out.

But the story freaked me out a little bit. Of all the things I had worried about, it had never once occurred to me that my kidney might be damaged during surgery—rendering it unable to help either Deb or me. That would have been such a terrible waste!

By the end of the day, my hospital room had begun to resemble Grand Central Station. Rabbi Werner stopped by on her chaplaincy rounds. We told her how much her welcoming Kol Nidre service had meant to us two weeks before, when we found ourselves "stranded" in Rochester over Yom Kippur. I had not thought seeing a chaplain would be important to us, but I was actually very glad to see her.

Margo, my donor advocate, and Lisa, my nurse transplant coordinator, also came by, as well as the social worker, a nutritionist, the on-call nephrologist, and other medical staff. I was presented with a fleece jacket with the Mayo Transplant Center logo and a certificate signed by the entire team: "Your gift brings with it the opportunity for renewed health and well-being and represents the highest form of generosity and compassion for others." They were very nice touches.

I did not sleep as well the second night. It was hard to find a comfortable position now, and I also kept needing to get up to pee. That pleased the nursing staff; it meant that my system was working. But getting in and out of bed was not easy. I could see the advantages of the catheter.

Even so, I was feeling pretty perky by the time Don arrived the next morning. It appeared two nights in the hospital were going to be sufficient. I hoped they would let me out.

All Systems Go

Journal entry by Martha Gershun—Sep 30, 2018

Well, all my bodily functions have returned (yay!), so I'm scheduled to leave the hospital after lunch. I've received extraordinary care here. Everyone is cheerful, courteous, and highly responsive to even the smallest request. On top of that, Don has taken terrific care of me—and his part of that work will continue when we transition back to the Marriott Residence Inn this afternoon. We took a stroll to visit Deb, her sister Barbie, and boyfriend George last night, and we'll visit again before lunch. Oh, and I get to take a shower after breakfast. Life is good!

Deb and I had decided on an adventure. On our last lunch together in Kansas City, she had given me a T-shirt with #Grateful emblazoned on the front. She had purchased a matching shirt, and we had agreed we would wear them for a photo op after our surgeries. Now we were ready. We both put on our shirts and set off down the halls looking for a good setting for a photograph. We found an empty corridor in front of some colorful Mayo artwork and posed while we made George, Don, and Barbie take numerous photos with their phones. We were determined to get a good shot to send to the *Jewish Chronicle*.

I was being released from the hospital, but Deb would be staying one more night before moving to the nearby condo where she would stay for several weeks while Mayo calibrated her postsurgery medication regimen.

While I started to pack up to leave, Don went to the hospital pharmacy to fill my prescription for OxyContin, as well as for extra-strength Tylenol. As promised, he had worked with the medical team to make sure I would have pain relief back at the hotel if I needed it. By midafternoon we had gone over all the post-op instructions and signed all the discharge paperwork. We were ready to make our escape.

I was very happy to settle on the living room couch in our hotel suite. Nathan and Bridget arrived from Minneapolis with bagels, flowers, and chocolates. It was wonderful to see them; their company was just what I needed.

The next four days were a weird mix of sleeping, watching TV, and a few brief outings. My Hawaii sister had emailed a gift card to a restaurant delivery service in Rochester, which turned out to be the perfect gift for a patient recovering from surgery in an out-of-town hotel. We ordered a lot of meals in. I never did need the Oxy, making do with the prescribed doses of Tylenol, and my pain decreased while my energy increased every day.

Tuesday night, we had a jolt when the fire alarm went off around nine. I might have been only four days post-op, but I believe very strongly in evacuating during fire alarms; it is part of my lifelong commitment to disaster preparedness. Despite Don's protests, I threw on my robe, grabbed my phone and my purse, and made him hustle with me down six flights of stairs. It was too cold to go outside, so the hotel patrons all huddled in the first floor lobby. We met a lovely woman who was there with her husband; she was scheduled to receive a kidney from her niece the next morning. She seemed very pleased to hear my strong accolades for the nurses on the Mayo transplant floor, and was relieved I was recovering so quickly; it boded well for her niece's donation procedure too. Eventually the fire department arrived, determined there was no actual threat, and turned off the alarm. The elevators still were not back online, so we walked back up the six flights to our hotel floor. Not bad for a convalescent, I thought.

By five days post-op, I felt well enough to walk the half mile with Don to the condo rental where Deb would be recuperating for the next several weeks. By now, both George and Barbie had left, and Deb's sister-in-law Carol had arrived from Kansas City to be her designated caregiver. Carol had gone to Pannekoeken for carryout, and we all enjoyed a delightful brunch of those amazing

Dutch pancakes. Deb had a long recovery path ahead, with an aggressive regimen of medications, infusions, tests, and medical appointments designed to prevent organ rejection. But, as always, she was taking everything in stride, spinning great yarns about their adventures navigating the Mayo subway with a wheelchair when a late-night procedure pushed them well past closing time.

On Thursday, six days post-op, I returned to Charlton 9 for my follow-up appointments. The physician's assistant reported that all looked good—I was healing on schedule. Lisa and I debriefed. She outlined my protocol going forward. Rest as needed, no lifting over ten pounds for four weeks, come back in four to six months for a full checkup to see how I was doing with just one kidney. The latter was optional, but an evaluation at Mayo paid for by Deb's insurance sounded like a good idea; I told Lisa we would be back. We hugged, and I headed out.

Leaving Mayo

It was dreary and rainy on Friday morning as we left the hotel. As I adjusted a pillow to protect my incision from the seat belt, I remembered Deb's admonition: "No matter what, buckle up on the way home. Even if it hurts. That's how I got my first kidney." Deb's first transplanted organs had been donated by the family of a middle-aged woman who had died in a car wreck; she had been lying down in the back without a seat belt. The woman was thrown from the car and died from the impact. When you are busy donating an organ as a living person, it is easy to forget how many organs come from generous families in the midst of great personal tragedy. In comparison, what I did felt easy.

Deb had asked us to swing by the condo where she was staying on our way out, and Carol ran out to hand me a package. It was a small box from Deb with a necklace inside. The pendant read, "I am Fearless."

As we drove out of Rochester toward the highway on-ramp I had the strangest feeling that I was leaving part of myself behind. I kept texting Deb to be sure she was still there. The whole point of this long, circuitous journey was to take out one of my organs and put it into her. We had started out as strangers, but now we were linked. Not in a creepy, stalky way, but in a profoundly loving way. We both entered into the same project with optimism and determination, and together we made it happen. We beat all the odds and got Deb a new lease on life. We made a miracle happen.

19

Follow-Up

(MARTHA)

Five months later, we were back on the road to Mayo for one final visit. I had been given a four-to-six-month window during which Deb's insurance company would pay for me to have a complete post-op evaluation.

My recovery had been uneventful. The first few days back home, close friends came over with coffee, bagels, salads, sushi, and, most importantly, good conversation. I was not in much pain, though I still was not driving, so those visits kept me from being isolated and bored. They also made me less dependent on Don, who really needed to get back to work.

The rest of the time, I slept. I had been warned that I would be tired after the surgery, but this overwhelming fatigue was different from anything I had ever experienced. It was not like the sleep deprivation after the birth of a child or the physical exhaustion after running a marathon. It was much gentler and much more pervasive, rolling in like fog, weighing me down with heavy, sodden clouds. Whether from the anesthesia, the trauma of surgery, or the sudden loss of 50 percent of my kidney function, this exhaustion was completely debilitating. Whatever I was doing, I had to sit down, then lie down, then sleep. It was also oddly comforting. I felt no guilt for turning down social invitations or meetings, unwilling to be far from home when the fog began to encroach. I was happy to stay home, manage small tasks, see friends for brief periods of time, and nap. At night, I slept more deeply than I had since I was a child.

The feeling was so pervasive that I idly wondered whether it would continue forever. On some level, I think I hoped it would. I had never given myself permission to be this undirected before. But, in fact, each day was a little clearer, and I began to regain my energy and my drive. Within the week, I was able to go with Don to a nearby friend's house for a fundraiser for our favored congressional candidate, an event John and I had worked together to help organize and promote. After several hours, I felt the fog on the edges of consciousness, and asked Don to usher me out and get me home before I crashed.

Two weeks after surgery, I sat on our deck and live-streamed a lecture from one of my favorite Harvard Business School professors, who was speaking at the reunion I was missing. That same day, I drove to our nearby village shopping center for lunch with a friend and then drove a few miles more to get my toenails done at the spa. I was mobile again!

The next week, I felt well enough to go to a hamburger joint to play Charity Drag Queen Bingo with my former colleagues at a fundraiser to support Jackson County CASA (Court Appointed Special Advocates). That was the first night that I really felt like myself again.

Four weeks after the surgery, I felt well enough to go with Don to New York City. I was able to visit friends and family, see two Broadway shows, eat at fabulous restaurants, and walk miles and miles of Manhattan streets.

I spent a lot of time on that trip with my freshman roommate, Perri. One afternoon, her son Orlando, a hospital-based psychiatrist in New York City, came over to his parents' apartment to visit. He speculated that donors like me are motivated by optimism, empathy, and a capacity for deferred gratification. Sounded right to me.

I was increasingly interested in the intellectual nuances of what I had done. I kept thinking about the oddity of having a part of myself now working inside someone else. This felt different from my gall bladder surgery several years before, when a diseased organ was removed from my body and discarded. And it was different from giving birth, when something had grown inside my body, become another distinct person, and then exited organically to live an independent life as a complete human being. This time an attached, healthy, functioning part of my body, my kidney, had been cut out of me and sewn inside someone else to continue its function—cleaning the blood of toxins—only now it was Deb's blood and Deb's toxins. There was something a little Frankenstein-like about knowing part of my body was doing its job inside someone else.

Sometime after Christmas, the fatigue finally abated for good, and the kidney adventure was no longer uppermost in my mind. If it had not been for the long scar down my belly, I could easily have forgotten anything had happened at all. By the time we were driving to Mayo for my checkup in late February, I cheerfully expected a pat on the back, hearty congratulations, and a pass to get on with my life.

Not surprisingly, there had been a couple of kerfluffles with the testing schedule for this trip. The scheduling team had booked the twenty-four-hour urine collection on the same day as the kidney function test, which was impossible—they either needed my pee in the orange jug, untainted, or they needed it marked with the radioactive contrast and deposited in the fake commode—they could not have it both ways. I got that straightened out by suggesting I do the twenty-four-hour collection on my drive up to Mayo, only to find the revised schedule they prepared left me no time to eat after my fasting blood draw and before the two-hour fast in advance of the kidney function test. So I got that changed too. Then two different boxes arrived from Mayo, each containing one of the large orange jugs and instructions for the twenty-four-hour collection. I emailed back again—no, I did not have to do the collection twice. It was just an error.

I had gotten good at managing the Mayo scheduling department and asking questions when things did not make sense. But after all the good feelings I was harboring about the excellent care I received after the transplant, I was sorry to be confronted again with their project management deficiencies.

Deb and I had stayed in touch through our recoveries, texting updates and funny stories. She had done much better than expected, recovering well and stabilizing quickly on her new immunosuppressant regimen. She progressed so rapidly she was able to leave Rochester a week early, returning to Florida just nineteen days after the transplant.

Now that we had both signed off CaringBridge, I followed Deb's progress on Facebook, where she posted beaming photos of her and George enjoying the Florida beach, concerts, restaurants, and community events. She looked terrific. Kidney recipients had a follow-up at Mayo too, and it turned out that Deb and I had booked our evaluations for the same week. She planned to leave just as we were arriving, but there would be one night's overlap. We made plans to meet for dinner.

Don and I got to the restaurant first (of course), and grabbed a quiet table near the back while we waited for Deb and George. I was excited to celebrate this anniversary together—five months post-op and doing great. Deb burst in, full of life, with George by her side. But before we picked up the menus she got very serious. After several days of tests, they had just met with the nephrologist for her wrap-up appointment. The news was mostly excellent: the swelling in Deb's legs and feet was gone, she was gaining weight, her incision looked perfect, and her labs were good—the kidney was filtering toxins and producing urine. At most medical centers, this would have been enough to declare Deb healthy and send her back home until the one-year checkup. But Mayo's routine midyear protocol included a kidney biopsy, considered the gold standard for detecting organ rejection. This more invasive, but more exacting, test can reveal signs of rejection at the cellular level, long before it shows up in lab work or through physical symptoms.

Deb's biopsy showed early signs of rejection, one of the worst things that can happen to an organ recipient. Fortunately, Mayo's hypervigilance allowed them to catch it early, so they could begin treatment before there was any damage to the kidney.

This news was a blow. Deb was very quick to tell me that the nephrologist said there was nothing either of us had done wrong. This had nothing to do with the health of my kidney starting out, and her compliance with the immunosuppression regimen had been letter perfect. I believed that. After all, Deb had kept her first kidney for twenty years, when the American Kidney Fund reports the average useful life of a cadaver kidney is fifteen years ("Deceased Donor Transplant" n.d.). She was good at this. Nonetheless, this time there was something wrong. Deb put up a brave front in the face of this tough news. While she and George were both clearly concerned about what this might mean for the long-term success of the transplant, they deflected by complaining about the inconvenience to their travel schedule instead. They had planned to fly home to Florida in the morning, clean bill of health in hand. Instead, they would now be staying another five days in Rochester while Deb received massive doses of IV prednisone on an outpatient basis. She could go home after that, on a reduced regimen of oral prednisone, but would have to return to Rochester in four weeks for another biopsy to see whether the inflammation had subsided. If the first-line treatment did not work, Mayo would move on to more aggressive interventions, most likely a central line for more powerful drugs. Deb said the nephrologist told her the midyear biopsy reveals early signs of rejection in 10 percent of kidney transplant cases.

Both Deb and George were determined to remain positive, and Don and I worked hard to follow their lead. Our dinner conversation was upbeat and wide-ranging—including news from Kansas City, reports on our families, politics, and vacation plans. Deb and George had a short cruise planned in a few weeks with Deb's college-age daughter—they were excited to be getting away after the ups and downs preceding the transplant and determined not to let this new setback interfere. We ate and drank and laughed a lot.

By the time dinner was over and Don and I were walking back to our hotel in the freezing Rochester winter, I was starting to fully process what Deb had told me. She was showing early signs of organ rejection. The transplant might be failing.

It was naïve, but up until that very moment I had given no serious consideration to this outcome. There had been so many hurdles leading up to the transplant that I had blithely assumed once we got that done and Deb and I had both survived the surgery, then everything would be fine. The Mayo website reported that 3 percent of living donor kidney transplants fail within one year, but those were very small numbers, and I truly never thought we would be one of those statistics. Even when the social workers had cautioned me during the donor evaluation process that not all kidney transplants are successful, I had paid no heed to their message.

I sorted through my feelings. I had worked very, very hard to get through the organ donation process. If her body rejected the kidney now, what would that mean about my effort and my sacrifice? Would that mean I had given up my kidney, and possibly compromised my own long-term health, for no good reason? Would this whole venture have been pointless? Would I have failed?

Don, as usual, was much more sanguine about the situation. We should wait and see what happened next before borrowing trouble. Mayo was the best clinic in the world. We should remain calm and positive and let them work their magic.

I felt like worrying would help.

But I had my own appointments to make and tests to take, and I was soon swept up once again in the Mayo machine. Early the next morning, I reported for my lab draws and turned in my twenty-four-hour urine collection. The tech reported that I had produced 25 percent more urine than the high end of the range. This implied good news about my kidney function. It also felt like vindication for a lifetime spent looking for the nearest bathroom. My mother used to joke that she could write a book about my childhood growing up in Southern California titled *Disneyland Potties I Have Known*. I truly was always the one who needed to stop to pee; maybe now I could stop apologizing.

The rest of the day was a mini version of my original three-day evaluation at Mayo. The last time, I had been very worried. This time it was just boring. I was no longer interested in the process or anxious about the results.

My meetings with Lisa, my nurse transplant coordinator, and Margo, my donor advocate, were like old home week. I was happy to deliver the good news that I had recovered quickly and felt well, like a star pupil delivering a straight A report card.

Lisa reminded me of the list of instructions to help ensure I had no long-term negative effects from giving up a kidney: drink lots of water, stay away from nonsteroidal anti-inflammatory drugs, or NSAIDs (like Advil), and see my primary care doctor annually to monitor my creatinine, urine protein, weight, and blood pressure. She also reminded me that one of the requirements to keep my "preferred status" on the United Network for Organ Sharing list if I needed a future transplant was to comply with the protocol to have my creatinine and urine protein tested at Mayo at both one and two years after organ donation. I did not have to come up again for the tests; I could just ship the samples to the lab. She also urged me to inform all future health care providers that I had donated a kidney so they could manage my care accordingly.

I told Lisa about Deb's biopsy results and asked her to explain what they meant. This happens sometimes, she said, it is why Mayo does early biopsies as part of their protocol. Mayo is very good at figuring out the right medication regimen to stop the rejection. There is no reason to be overly concerned. She was also very clear in her directions to me: You have given your kidney away; your responsibility is over.

Since Deb and George were still stuck in Rochester for the prednisone infusions, they came over to our hotel to visit. Deb also wanted to deliver several bags of winter clothes that she had brought for the Minnesota cold, but did not need to take back to sunny Florida. Don and I had agreed to drive the bags back home to Kansas City; I would take them over to Deb's parents' house when we got home.

The next morning I dropped the blood pressure gear off at the desk on Charlton 10 and waited to talk with the nephrology and hypertension nurse about the results. She had good news. My eighteen-hour blood pressures were in the normal range, averaging 122/71. In fact, my readings in the office were fairly low: 102/62. For the first time in my life, I was warned to watch for the symptoms of low blood pressure and what to do if they should occur.

The nurse also had portal access to the rest of my tests. She was particularly pleased that my creatinine looked good—1.22 mg/dL, which is high for an adult female (normal range is 0.59–1.04), but excellent for someone with only one kidney, where normal could be 1.8 or 1.9. My twenty-four-hour protein was 151 mg, which was very good, and my corrected iothalamate GFR (glomerular filtration rate) from that weird kidney function test was 71. That was particularly reassuring, since the normal range for someone with two working kidneys is 66–120. The nurse pointed to that result: "Your remaining kidney is doing great. In fact, someone with these numbers and two kidneys could be approved to donate." Her overall assessment: I had very strong kidney function to start with, and my remaining kidney was pulling the load now that it was alone.

My last scheduled appointment was with yet another nephrologist, Dr. Lorenz, who would provide my final sign-off. I was a little disappointed that Dr. Bentall was not on the rotation that day. I would have liked to have seen him at the end of this journey. As it turned out, I barely got to even see Dr. Lorenz. Instead, most of my appointment time was spent with a nephrology fellow, clearly assigned to meet with the patients who had nothing wrong with them. He reviewed my labs and numbers again and gave me much the same advice I had been hearing all along—drink lots of water, avoid NSAIDs, keep exercising, lose weight. He was also the first person to tell me that radioactive contrast material can damage kidneys; he cautioned me not to agree to its use in future tests without careful discussion with the ordering physician. I found that ironic since they had just used that material in the kidney function test. I guess that had been an exception.

At the very end of our consultation, Dr. Lorenz came in. She quickly reviewed the fellow's notes, shook my hand, thanked me for my service, and sent us on our way. I was relieved that there was not much to talk about. But it still felt anticlimactic after everything I had been through. I had somehow expected more.

A Living Saint

While the doctors at Mayo might treat organ donors like ordinary patients without interesting health problems, other people in my life definitely did not. On the one hand, I appreciated those who acknowledged the recent adventure that had dominated my life for much of a year. On the other hand, I was very uncomfortable when people idealized my actions, hailing me as a hero or a living saint. One of my college roommates, now a Lutheran minister, suggested that putting living organ donors on a pedestal was one way people dealt with their own discomfort about not volunteering to do something like this. She described their theoretical reasoning this way: "I know I'm not a saint. So if only saints do this, then I don't have to think about doing it."

I thought the same was possibly true with people's reaction to my quick recovery. When I would see people out in the community, even months after the surgery, they would fawn over me: "How are you?" they would ask with great concern, very solicitous. Often they seemed slightly disappointed when I would say, "Just fine, thanks. I feel like it never happened at all." I began to think people wanted organ donation to have consequences. If it was too easy, then maybe everyone should consider it.

I thought about it differently. In my worldview, everyone has their own mitzvot to perform—whether they donate money or volunteer time to a nonprofit or help their neighbors or pursue a career in public service. Donating a kidney happened to be one of mine.

I also knew a lot of ways I was far from heroic. I am so claustrophobic I do not park in underground parking lots; I could never go into a cave to save a stranger. I am terrified of drowning; even though I am an excellent swimmer, I do not think I could dive into a lake to free someone from a submerged car. For nearly eight years I worked at Jackson County CASA, helping abused and neglected children, and never once did I seriously think about adopting—or even fostering—a child in desperate need of a home.

Those weren't mitzvot I could do. But I could do this. I am not squeamish about needles or hospitals. I was retired, so I had the time. I had the support system, especially Don's willingness and ability to serve as my caregiver. This mitzvah also seemed finite to me. Unlike adopting a child out of the system—a good deed that has lifelong implications—donating a kidney was a very intense mitzvah over a very defined period of time. After the donation was over, my life essentially returned to normal.

I also thought a lot about what it meant to be one of the very few people in this country to donate a kidney to a stranger. By my count, Don and I together spent more than 380 hours, or nearly ten full work weeks, to ensure this kidney transplant was successful. Our out-of-pocket costs, including those that Deb reimbursed, were more than $4,000. This is a huge burden to place on donors and their families, in addition to the actual risk and effort of the transplant surgery. It was easy to see that not everyone could manage that burden.

I also came to better understand how living organ donors' unique place in the medical system made the process so frustrating: we are part supply chain component and part patient, all at the same time. While I assumed Mayo had excellent systems for managing their supply chain—drugs, supplies, equipment—and they clearly had excellent systems for managing their patients, they had no integrated system for managing a person who was both. For someone like me—with a business education and managerial experience, high customer service standards, and a low tolerance for uncertainty and delay—this ambiguity was maddening. Surely there were better ways to manage living donors if the system was serious about enlarging that pool to meet the demand for much-needed organs. One of my favorite Harvard Business School professors, Ben Shapiro, had written an article years ago titled "Staple Yourself to an Order" that argued that senior executives should take the time to track every step of an order management process so they would understand the customer's experience at every stage in the cycle (Shapiro, Rangan, and Svikola 2004). I came to believe that if transplant centers considered every part of the transplant process from the living donor's perspective, they would see many opportunities for improvement. I bet these improvements would increase the number of people able and willing to donate, as well as retaining more volunteers all the way through to the actual transplant surgery.

I spent the weeks after we returned from Mayo stalking Deb on Facebook. I saw when she completed the prednisone regimen at Mayo and returned home to Florida to wait out the remaining three weeks before the second biopsy. Her Facebook page began to show fabulous photos of the planned post-op cruise—dazzling sunshine, calm blue seas, mouthwatering food, swimming with dolphins, Mayan ruins, and, most astounding of all, video of Deb zip-lining in Honduras. Now that was definitely something my kidney would never have gotten to do before the transplant!

By March 13, Deb was back in Rochester for another kidney biopsy. The next day, we finally got the news we had been waiting for. She texted, "no sign of rejection, and the inflammation is almost gone." No more extraordinary treatment was necessary. Mayo's aggressive early intervention had worked.

With my health confirmed and Deb's health recovered, the project felt completed. All that remained were a few residual signs that something very important had occurred once upon a time. I would return to my "normal life," but I would always have the scar down my belly and always be on alert for news of Deb's well-being. I would focus more on my own nutrition and exercise routine and check my blood pressure daily. I would proudly put "Living Organ Donor" on my Twitter and Facebook profiles, and volunteer to talk to prospective donors and recipients who might like to hear about someone's firsthand experience with the system. Deb and I would speak together at my synagogue about what organ donation meant to us, and we would continue to look for more opportunities to present together. I would join the local advisory board of the National Kidney Foundation. And, of course, I would partner with John to write this book.

Donating a kidney was one of the most profoundly meaningful experiences of my life. It was frustrating and difficult and annoying and scary. It was also exciting and joyous and deeply rewarding.

If I could, I would do it again.

20

Lessons Learned

(JOHN)

One of the key lessons learned from Martha's story is that kidney donors are not patients in the traditional sense of that word. They are not sick. They do not need to see a doctor. They do not need surgery. They are altruistically volunteering to undergo a painful and potentially dangerous procedure to benefit another person. Instead of thinking of them as patients, we should perhaps think of them as philanthropists. They are philanthropists who donate a body part instead of donating money.

Transplant centers do not treat organ donors like philanthropists. If they did, they would provide every possible support for the donor's efforts. They would cultivate donors by showing gratitude and publicly acknowledging the donor's generosity. Instead, they make the process of donation unaccountably difficult.

Until transplant centers change their attitudes, their procedures and practices, and their ethos with regard to living donors, many people who otherwise might be good candidates to donate will not be willing or able or motivated to do so. We have no idea how many people are out there who are willing and perhaps even eager to donate but are put off by the process or the cost. We do not know how many people start the process of being evaluated as a donor and then drop out because of the sorts of barriers that

Martha so eloquently describes. We cannot afford to lose those donors.

We can learn a couple of other key lessons from Martha's experience as a living unrelated donor. The most obvious is also the easiest to take for granted: the transplant worked. The fact that an unrelated donor can safely give a kidney and that it can successfully engraft and function is astounding. It is also increasingly commonplace. People can successfully donate kidneys to somebody to whom they are totally unrelated.

The fact that transplants from living donors are usually successful means that, collectively, we could completely eliminate the waiting list for organ transplants. There are about one hundred thousand people on the waiting list for a kidney transplant in the United States. There are 330 million people in the United States. If one of every thousand of us offered to donate, as Martha did, and even if only one-third of those generous volunteers were deemed eligible and found a matching recipient, then everybody on the current waiting list would get a kidney.

This would keep many from needing to begin burdensome dialysis treatments, as well as helping those who now survive only by undergoing dialysis while waiting for a cadaveric donor. Many die waiting. Increasing the pool of living donors would decrease long waits for a kidney, thus saving many people who die before receiving an organ. It would also lead to better outcomes than those experienced following deceased donor transplants. Five-year survival for patients who get a kidney from a living donor is 94 percent. For those who get a cadaveric kidney, it is 87 percent (Hart et al. 2017). Within ten years, half of cadaveric kidneys fail compared to one-third of kidneys from living donors.

Increasing the number of kidney transplants is good for society too. Not only are the medical outcomes better but the costs are lower than keeping a patient on dialysis. Different studies estimate the cost savings slightly differently. But all agree that kidney transplants are more cost-effective in the long run than dialysis. According to a recent report by the University of California San Francisco, dialysis in the United States costs an average of $89,000 per year, while the average cost of a kidney transplant is $32,000 for the transplant surgery and $25,000 per year after surgery to care for the patient and ensure the transplant is not rejected. The costs of posttransplant care get even lower in subsequent years, while the cost of dialysis remains constant.

These cost savings are passed on directly to the American people. Dialysis and transplantation are both covered by private insurance. For those who are uninsured, they are paid for by the federal Medicare program, regardless of the patient's age. The program pays for the care of over half a million people every year, and the number is growing. Today, Medicare coverage for kidney patients costs over $35 billion annually, approximately 6 percent of all Medicare expenditures. As the *Economist* noted on February 20, 2020, it is estimated that every kidney transplant for a patient without private insurance generates about $150,000 in Medicare savings for US taxpayers ("Kidney Failure"). As one academic review put it, "Compared with dialysis, kidney transplantation leads to improved patient survival and quality of life, as well as cost savings to the health payer" (Klarenbach, Barnieh, and Gill 2009, 534).

If more people like Martha were willing to donate a kidney, lives and money would be saved. Alas, the sort of generosity that Martha showed is rare. Since kidney transplantation started in the 1950s, about fifty thousand living people have donated kidneys, according to the National Kidney Registry ("Living Donors n.d.). Today, about 1,000–1,500 people donate each year to an unrelated person. Another three thousand donate to a family member. Most people are not as altruistic as Martha. Most people would never undergo a nephrectomy to help a stranger. But eliminating barriers and costs might help.

There are efforts to mitigate some of these obstacles. The paired donations and voucher programs that we discussed eliminate the barriers that are associated with biology. They overcome histocompatibility problems and allow people to help a loved one, even if the loved one does not get a kidney directly from a family member.

Transplant centers have also eliminated some of the barriers caused by suspicion of the motives of people who want to donate to a stranger. We have learned that there are different types of altruism. The altruism of a family member donating to a loved one is different from the altruism of a person who donates to a stranger (Seelig and Rosof 2001). In many ways, family members are less altruistic, since they presumably derive some psychological benefit from saving a loved one. Family members may also be more subject to subtle (or overt) coercion from the recipient or other family members. These considerations suggest the bar should be higher in terms of evaluating voluntariness among potential family donors than among people who choose to donate to a stranger. Strangers' motivations may be difficult to understand, but they are unlikely to feel psychological pressure from family members to donate. If anything, the opposite is likely to be true: family members and friends may discourage such donors, as I initially did with Martha.

In assessing the motivations of donors, transplant centers have sought a delicate balance. They screen donors for obvious psychopathology. They try to ascertain whether there is coercion. They look for conditions that might indicate a higher-than-normal psychological risk, such as mood disorders or substance abuse. But they seldom probe deeper to understand the true underlying motivations of donors. As Martha's narrative makes clear, those underlying motivations may be complex, quite personal, and impossible to rank on a scale designed to predict the risk of a bad psychological outcomes. Still, we try.

Research into the motivations of donors led to the development and widespread adoption of a set of guidelines for evaluating stranger donors. The guidelines were based on identifying factors that either increased or decreased the risk of bad psychological outcomes for donors. Donors are considered to be at higher risk of a bad outcome if they have an underlying psychiatric disorder, if they have substance abuse, lack health insurance, or have limited cognitive capacity, multiple family stressors, poor family support, unrealistic expectations, or ambivalence about donating. They are at low risk if they have none of those findings. The guidelines concluded by saying, "The safety and well-being of each donor will be maximized only by considering (a) the unique circumstances that led the individual to come forward for donation and (b) the unique set of psychosocial risk and protective factors that the individual brings" (Dew et al. 2007, 1051).

Alison Heru, a psychologist in Colorado, noted, "The ideal low risk non-directed donor is described in the Guidelines as a person who has a stable life with no recent significant losses/ stressors, has the support of their family, financial resources, and has a history of medical altruism" (Heru 2018, 1). In some cases, like Martha's, these donors come to know the recipient. In others, the donor and recipient never meet, because one or both choose to remain anonymous.

Sometimes, we find psychopathological reasons for donation. Robert D. Truog, the Frances Glessner Lee Professor of Medical Ethics, Anesthesiology and Pediatrics at Harvard Medical School, where he is also the director of the Center for Bioethics, writes,

"The radical altruism that motivates a person to make a potentially life-threatening sacrifice for a stranger calls for careful scrutiny" (Truog 2005, 445). One recent case involved a man who seemed pathologically obsessed with giving away everything, from his money to his organs, saying that doing so was "as much a necessity as food, water, and air" (Parker 2004, 55). Truog concluded that, because of such cases, "transplantation teams have an obligation to assess potential donors in all these dimensions and prohibit donations that arouse serious concern" (Truog 2005, 446).

Many transplant centers and advocacy organizations now encourage, train, and help patients to "recruit" unrelated donors using conventional and social media, personal networks, and other resources. Some hospitals, such as the University of Pittsburgh Medical Center and the University of Alabama at Birmingham, have initiated Living Donor Champion programs, where patients recruit an advocate, or champion, to help them find a living donor. Pittsburgh even launched its own television ad campaign, encouraging people more broadly to consider becoming living donors.

The National Kidney Foundation has a program called The Big Ask: The Big Give. On their website, they have many videos telling the stories of donors and recipients. The American Transplant Foundation coaches patients on how to "crowdsource for an organ" (Medaris Miller n.d.). People who need kidneys put signs in their front yards, wear T-shirts, put up posters, and place decals on their cars advertising their need. All these efforts attempt to increase the number of living organ donors.

Social media is providing even more innovative ways to help people reach potential donors. A Facebook app called Donor was developed to direct the patient's initial appeal to friends and family, where it was most likely to be effective (Bramstedt and Cameron 2017). There is now even a smartphone app for publicizing the need for a kidney (Kumar et al. 2016). An article in the *New York Daily News* recounted how April Capone, former mayor of East Haven, Connecticut, saw a post pop up in her Facebook feed. A resident of her city, Carlos, was at Mayo, waiting for a kidney. Capone volunteered to donate. She later said, "I knew from the second I saw his post that I was going to be a donor." Capone said she had no personal reason for donating a kidney; she just want to save a life. "It was the best thing I ever did with my life," she said. "I wish I had more; I would do it again" (Associated Press 2012).

The use of social media to seek donors raises interesting questions about equality. Access to social media, like access to all internet services, is not equally distributed. It is highly associated with household income. Thus, patients with more income will be more likely to advertise on social media and more likely to get kidneys. The dilemma is a familiar one. On the one hand, increasing the number of people who donate will be good for everyone. Even poor patients who cannot themselves advertise would benefit if a wealthier person who was ahead of them on the waiting list for a transplant received an organ that was procured through a social media campaign. But, while everyone would be better-off, some would be disproportionately more well-off. Disparities would be exacerbated. The alternative, though, is to let everybody be worse off, but equally worse off.

Such advertising, whether through conventional or social media, is completely legal, although offering money for donations is not. Some have expressed skepticism about the ethics of advertising. The skepticism arises out of fear that ads could contain misleading information, be emotionally manipulative, and lead to preferential allocation of organs to people who are more attractive or whose story is more compelling (Baboolal 2018, 1405–6).

Although the shift to encourage living organ donation is under-way, it is far from complete. Martha's tale illustrates in excruciating detail what it is like for potential donors still experiencing the slow, steady transition from discouragement (or prohibition) to accep-tance and encouragement of such altruistic acts.

The existence of a program like the one at Mayo (and many other medical centers around the country) that accepts unrelated donors illustrates two things. One is the remarkable medical and moral triumphs that make such transplantation safe and success-ful. Scientists, clinicians, and administrators have built extraordi-nary systems to enable somebody to safely donate a kidney to a stranger. Such systems require careful medical and psychosocial screening of the donor, sophisticated immunological match-ing of donor and recipient, coordinated timing of the donation and transplant operations, and meticulous postoperative care, as well as lifetime immunosuppressant management for the recipi-ent. Both donor and recipient must receive the psychological and spiritual support they need. Ethical and legal considerations must be addressed. There must be a way to finance these complex opera-tions, as well as the medical and psychological workups necessary for donor and recipient evaluation, and the follow-up care that both will require. In the story of Martha and Deb, all those systems worked. Deb's transplant was successful.

Another way to read the tale is the story of a system that is outdated and inefficient, that discourages stranger donors and makes their lives frustrating and inconvenient. The system does not smooth the logistics for donors to get evaluated or comply with necessary post-op requirements. It does not have a system-atic way to reimburse donors and their caregivers for the out-of-pocket costs for travel or time off work for evaluation, surgery, and recovery. As one study notes, "Although the donation process should be financially neutral, living kidney donors may experience out-of-pocket expenses and lost wages that may or may not be completely covered through regional or national reimbursement programs, and may face difficulties arranging subsequent life and health insurance" (Lentine, Lam, and Segey 2019, 601).

Furthermore, protocols to keep prospective donors informed, sustained, and encouraged during the lengthy process of evaluation and the waiting period until surgery are often inadequate. The good outcome in Martha and Deb's case depended on the careful medical evaluation at Mayo, but it also required extraordinary dedication and energy from Martha herself to figure out what was required and how to get it done. Martha persevered despite the costs and the strangely unhelpful glitches she encountered. Not all potential donors would do the same.

As the number of stranger donors has steadily increased, doctors have continued to learn better ways to predict which donations will be safe for the donor and successful for the recipient. The process at Mayo that Martha experienced exemplifies that focus on safety. Their careful attention to Martha's blood pressure and blood sugar numbers illustrates this. In both cases, she was almost rejected as a donor because her blood pressure and blood sugar were ever so slightly outside normal ranges (and, as it turned out, her blood sugar was probably not outside that range at all). Both hypertension and diabetes can cause kidney problems. A person with just one kidney is obviously at higher risk for a bad outcome from kidney disease caused by those conditions than a person with two kidneys. Mayo's decision-making algorithm, like similar ones at most transplant centers, was based on the idea that they would rather forgo a potentially lifesaving kidney donation than take even the slightest risk that the donor could develop problems.

The same risk aversion holds true for their psychological criteria. When they found out, through Martha's own admission, that she had seen a mental health professional in the past, they demanded to see all Martha's therapy records. This demand not only seemed absurdly intrusive but also seemed to reflect the sort of suspicion that unrelated donors must be irrational. As it turned out, Mayo was willing to bend the criteria and accept a summary from Martha's therapist. But why go there at all, especially since the transplant program does its own evaluation of the mental health of potential donors?

These risk thresholds are ethical choices, not scientific ones. Had Martha's blood pressure stayed elevated, or had medication failed to control it, she probably would still have been fine after donation. That is, the odds that mild hypertension would end up causing her health problems over the remaining duration of her life were low. Still, the odds were slightly higher than if she had two kidneys. And that slight tilting of the scales would have been enough for Mayo to send her packing and tell Deb that the search for an appropriate donor must resume.

Mayo's choice is not the only defensible ethical choice. A different approach would be less paternalistic—that is, less certain that medical professionals knew what was best for the donor, even if the donor disagreed—and more willing to defer to the donor's autonomy and a process of informed consent. By that approach, Mayo clinicians would have conveyed their findings to Martha and explained the risks of hypertension or high blood sugar for someone with only one kidney. Once they were convinced that she understood the risks, and once they concluded that she was not being coerced, then they would have left the decision about whether to proceed up to her. Instead, they held the final say about whether or not she would be accepted as a donor. They reserved the right to say whether they would take the risk of allowing her to take certain risks.

The relevance of marijuana use displays a similar paternalism, though, in that case, it is less clear which specific risks members of the transplant team were concerned about. Were they worried that marijuana was the tip of the iceberg, and that, if Martha occasionally smoked pot then she also might use heroin or other injectable drugs? Was the concern that such hypothetical IV drug use might make her more likely to carry hepatitis or some other transmissible disease? Or were they concerned that using pot was a psychological red flag, indicating a fragile psyche for which Martha was "self-medicating"? Perhaps they were worried that, if Deb did not do well, Martha would tailspin into a serious depression or more serious drug use. If all recreational marijuana users need to fear they will be rejected as organ donors, there will be a lot fewer people stepping up to volunteer.

As the need for transplantable organs grows, we should, by policy, be encouraging donation, making the process easier and more convenient, and deferring more to donors as the proper assessors of the appropriate risk threshold.

Ultimately, efforts to increase the number of stranger donors will only succeed if society learns to regard such donations as a legitimate process and one that ought to be facilitated rather than hampered, and encouraged rather than discouraged.

A few relatively straightforward changes might improve donation rates.

First, programs for living donors should adopt a model similar to that of Belfast City Hospital and implement a donor evaluation process that can be done in a day. It is possible. It just takes planning and an institutional commitment.

Second, the reasonable costs to donors and their caregivers of both evaluation and surgery, including travel costs and the cost of time off work, should be reimbursed by the recipients' insurance or by Medicare for the uninsured. After all, it is the insurance company, or Medicare, that saves money every time a patient on dialysis receives a successful kidney transplant. Why should living donors subsidize that savings out of their own pockets in addition to donating their organs?

It should be apparent from my conclusions that my own views about kidney donation to a stranger have changed as a result of going through this adventure with my friend Martha. I was deeply moved by her experiences. At the outset, I tried to discourage her and worried that she was underestimating the risks or burdens of the procedure. Today, I think that I was overestimating them. I always knew that kidney donation was an act of extraordinary generosity. I learned, too, that we have not yet developed the societal mechanisms, or the proper procedures within health care institutions, to honor that generosity in the ways that it deserves to be honored. We can do better. We need to find ways to make donation less costly, less time-consuming, and less intrusive. If we do, we will harness the altruism that is out there and save many lives.

Epilogue

September 1, 2020

It has now been nearly two years since Martha donated her kidney to Deb at the Mayo Clinic in Rochester. Both women continue to enjoy good health, with no significant complications from the procedure. Like all transplant recipients, Deb continues to follow a strict regimen of immunosuppressant medications to "trick" her body into accepting the organ that came from someone else. Because these medications put transplant recipients at particular risk for COVID-19, she has been especially vigilant throughout the pandemic. She also continues to return to Mayo for periodic checkups. The sixth-month follow-up was Martha's last visit to the clinic. One year after the donation surgery, Mayo sent her a lab kit to collect urine and blood samples to return for testing. Fortunately, it did not require dry ice. Those tests showed that Martha continued to do well with one kidney. She just received another lab kit from Mayo to return at the second anniversary of her donation surgery. After that, she will follow up with her primary care physician on her regular schedule.

Martha and Deb stay in contact using Facebook, texts, and occasional phone calls. Before the pandemic they periodically found time to get together for lunch when Deb came to Kansas City to visit her family. Deb also encouraged Martha to come visit her and George in Fort Lauderdale, a trip they all hope will be safe again sometime soon. Whenever they talk, their raucous conversation is filled with updates, stories, and lots of laughter. They both look forward to a future filled with many years of health, happiness, and friendship.

Resources

The following organizations provide information about organ transplants for both donors and recipients:

American Kidney Fund
https://www.kidneyfund.org

American Liver Foundation
https://www.liverfoundation.org

American Transplant Foundation
https://www.americantransplantfoundation.org

The Division of Transplantation, US Department of Health and
    Human Services
https://www.organdonor.gov

Donate Life America
https://www.donatelife.net

Living Kidney Donors Network
http://www.lkdn.org

National Foundation for Transplants
https://www.transplants.org

National Kidney Foundation
https://www.kidney.org

National Kidney Registry
https://www.kidneyregistry.org

National Living Donor Assistance Center
https://www.livingdonorassistance.org

Organ Procurement and Transplantation Network, US Department of Health and Human Services
https://optn.transplant.hrsa.gov

Renewal
https://www.renewal.org

United Network for Organ Sharing
https://www.unos.org

Works Cited

Ahmad, M. Usman, Afif Hanna, Ahmed-Zayn Mohamed, Alex Schlindwein, Caitlin Pley, Ingrid Bahner, Rahul Suresh Mhaskar, Gavin J. Pettigrew, and Tambi Jarmi. 2019. "A Systematic Review of Opt-Out versus Opt-In Consent on Deceased Organ Donation and Transplantation (2006–2016)." *World Journal of Surgery* 43 (12): 3161–71. https://doi.org/10.1007/s00268-019-05118-4.

Allard, Julie, Aviva Goldberg, and Marie-Chantal Fortin. 2014. "Regulated Markets of Kidneys in Developed Countries or How to Increase Health Inequities." *American Journal of Bioethics* 14 (10): 44–45. https://doi.org/10.1080/15265161.2014.947442.

"April Is Donate Life Month." 2018. *Kansas City Jewish Chronicle*. April 19, 2018. https://kcjc.com/index.php/current-news/latest-news/4843-lp04-19-18.

Associated Press. 2012. "Facebook Now a Great Way to Find a Kidney: Organ Donations Matched through Social Media on the Rise." *New York Daily News*, January 2, 2012. https://www.nydailynews.com/life-style/health/facebook-great-find-kidney-organ-donations-matched-social-media-rise-article-1.999851.

Aviv, Rachel. 2018. "What Does It Mean to Die?" *New Yorker*, January 29, 2018. https://www.newyorker.com/magazine/2018/02/05/what-does-it-mean-to-die.

Axelrod, David, Mark A. Schnitzler, Huiling Xiao, Abhijit S. Naik, Dorry L. Segev, Vikas R. Dharnidharka, Daniel C. Brennan, and Krista L. Lentine. 2017. "The Changing Financial Landscape of Renal Transplant Practice: A National Cohort Analysis." *American Journal of Transplantation* 17 (2): 377–89. https://doi.org/10.1111/ajt.14018.

Baboolal, Kesh. 2018. "Crowdsourcing for Organs: A Social Dilemma." *Transplantation* 102 (9): 1405–6. https://doi.org/10.1097/TP.0000000000002210.

"The Big Ask: The Big Give." n.d. National Kidney Foundation. Accessed March 17, 2020. https://www.kidney.org/transplantation/livingdonors.

"Blood Tests for Transplant." n.d. National Kidney Foundation. Accessed March 17, 2020. https://www.kidney.org/atoz/content/BloodTests-for-Transplant.

Boas, Hagi. 2011. "Where Do Human Organs Come From? Trends in Generalized and Restricted Altruism in Organ Donations." *Social Science & Medicine* 73:1378–85. https://doi.org/10.1016/j.socscimed.2011.07.028.

Borschel, Amanda. 2015. "Arizona Rabbi Donates His 'Spare' Kidney to Save Young Israeli." *Times of Israel*, June 19, 2015. https://www.timesofisrael.com/arizona-rabbi-donates-his-spare-kidney-to-save-young-israeli/.

Boudville, Neil, G. V. Ramesh Prasad, Greg Knoll, Norman Muirhead, Heather Thiessen-Philbrook, Robert C. Yang, M. Patricia Rosas-Arellano, Abdulrahman Housawi, and Amit X. Garg. 2006. "Meta-Analysis: Risk for Hypertension in Living Kidney Donors." *Annals of Internal Medicine* 145 (3): 185–96. https://doi.org/10.7326/0003-4819-145-3-200608010-00006.

Boyarsky, Brian J., Teresa Po-Yu Chiang, William A. Werbel, Christine M. Durand, Robin K. Avery, Samantha N. Getsin, Kyle R. Jackson, et al. 2020. "Early Impact of COVID-19 on Transplant Center Practices and Policies in the United States. *American Journal of Transplantation* 20 (7): 1809–18. https://doi.org/10.1111/ajt.15915.

Bramstedt, Katrina A., and Andrew MacGregor Cameron. 2017. "Beyond the Billboard: The Facebook-Based Application, Donor, and Its Guided Approach to Facilitating Living Organ Donation." *American Journal of Transplantation* 17 (2): 336–40. https://doi.org/10.1111/ajt.14004.

Calne, Roy. 2008. "Early Days of Liver Transplantation." *American J. of Transplantation* 8 (9): 1775–78. https://doi.org/10.1111/j.1600-6143.2008.02315.x.

Calne, Roy, Kirk Rolles, Sathia Thiru, P. Mcmaster, G. N. Craddock, S. Aziz, Douglas J. White, et al. 1979. "Cyclosporin A Initially as the Only Immunosuppressant in 34 Recipients of Cadaveric Organs: 32 Kidneys, 2 Pancreases, and 2 Livers." *Lancet* 314 (8151): 1033–36. https://doi.org/10.1016/s0140-6736(79)92440-1.

Cherry, Mark J. 2017. "Organ Vouchers and Barter Markets: Saving Lives, Reducing Suffering, and Trading in Human Organs." *Journal of Medicine & Philosophy* 42 (5): 503–17. https://doi.org/10.1093/jmp/jhx019.

Cronin, Antonia J., and David Price. 2008. "Directed Organ Donation: Is the Donor the Owner?" *Clinical Ethics* 3 (3): 127–31. https://doi.org/10.1258/ce.2008.008018.

"Current State of Organ Donation and Transplantation." 2020. Data. United Network for Organ Sharing. Accessed Aug. 25, 2020. https://unos.org/covid/.

"Deceased Donor Transplant." n.d. American Kidney Fund. Accessed March 17, 2020. https://www.kidneyfund.org/kidney-disease/kidney-failure/treatment-of-kidney-failure/kidney-transplant/deceased-donor-transplant.html.

Dew, Mary Amanda, C. L. Jacobs, Sheila G. Jowsey, Ruthanne L. Hanto, Charles Miller, Francis L. Delmonico. 2007. "Guidelines for the Psychosocial Evaluation of Living Unrelated Kidney Donors in the United States." *American Journal of Transplantation* 7 (5): 1047–54. https://doi.org/10.1111/j.1600–6143.2007.01751.x.

Dorflinger, Lindsey M., Sanjay Kulkarni, Carrie Thiessen, Sharon Klarman, and Liana Fraenkel. 2018. "Assessing Living Donor Priorities through Nominal Group Technique." *Progress in Transplantation* 28 (1): 29–35. https://doi.org/10.1177/1526924817746682.

"Eligibility Guidelines." n.d. National Living Donor Assistance Center. Accessed March 17, 2020. https://www.livingdonorassistance.org/How-to-Apply/Eligibility-Guidelines.

Formica, Richard N., Jr. 2017. "A Critical Assessment on Kidney Allocation Systems." Abstract. *Transplantation Reviews* 31, no. 1. https://doi.org/10.1016/j.trre.2016.10.002.

Fox, Renée, and Judith Swazey. 1974. *The Courage to Fail*. Chicago: University of Chicago Press.

Garg, Amit X., G. V. Ramesh Prasad, Heather R. Thiessen-Philbrook, Li Ping, Magda Melo, Eric M. Gibney, Greg Knoll, et al. 2008. "Cardiovascular Disease and Hypertension Risk in Living Kidney Donors: An Analysis of Health Administrative Data in Ontario, Canada." *Transplantation* 86 (3): 399–406. https://doi.org/10.1097/TP.0b013e31817ba9e3.

Gibney, Eric M., Anne L. King, Daniel G. Maluf, Amit Garg, and Chirag Parikh. 2007. "Living Kidney Donors Requiring Transplantation: Focus on African Americans." *Transplantation* 84 (5): 647–49. https://doi.org/10.1097/01.tp.0000277288.78771.c2.

Gill, Jagbir, James Dong, Caren Rose, Olwyn Johnston, David Landsberg, and John Gill. 2013. "The Effect of Race and Income on Living Kidney Donation in the United States." *Journal of the American Society of Nephrology* 24 (11): 1872–79. https://doi.org/10.1681/ASN.2013010049.

"Giving of Oneself: Member of the Kansas City Jewish Community in Search of a New Kidney." 2017. *Kansas City Jewish Chronicle*. December 28, 2017. http://www.kcjc.com/current-news/latest-news/4667-giving-of-oneself-member-of-the-kansas-city-jewish-community-in-search-of-a-new-kidney.

Graham, Judi M., and Aisling E. Courtney. 2018. "The Adoption of a One-Day Donor Assessment Model in a Living Kidney Donor Transplant Program:

A Quality Improvement Project." *American Journal of Kidney Disease* 71 (2): 209–15. https://doi.org/10.1053/j.ajkd.2017.07.013.

Hart, Allyson, Jodi Marie Smith, Melissa A. Skeans, Sally K. Gustafson, Darren E. Stewart, Wida S. Cherikh, Jennifer L. Wainright, et al. 2017. "OPTN/SRTR 2015 Annual Data Report: Kidney." *American Journal of Transplantation* 17 (Suppl. 1): 21–116. https://doi.org/10.1111/ajt.14124.

Heru, Alison. 2018. "Should Narrative Coherence Be Considered in the Assessment of Motivation in the Non-Directed Kidney Donation?" *General Hospital Psychiatry* 55:1–3. https://doi.org/10.1016/j.genhosppsych.2018.08.005.

"HHS Launches President Trump's 'Advancing American Kidney Health' Initiative." 2019. Press release. US Department of Health and Human Services. July 10, 2019. https://www.hhs.gov/about/news/2019/07/10/hhs-launches-president-trump-advancing-american-kidney-health-initiative.html.

Hippen, Benjamin. 2005. "In Defense of a Regulated Market in Kidney from Living Vendors." *Journal of Medicine & Philosophy* 30 (6): 593–626. https://doi.org/10.1080/03605310500421397.

"How Can I Find a Living Donor?" n.d. University of Pittsburgh Medical Center Transplant Services. Accessed March 17, 2020. https://www.upmc.com/services/transplant/liver/living-donor/find-a-living-donor.

HRSA (Health Resources and Services Administration). n.d. "What Can Be Donated." US Government Information on Organ Donation and Transplantation. Accessed March 17, 2020. https://www.organdonor.gov/about/what.html.

iSpot.tv. 2018. UPMC TV Commercial, "Living Donor Liver Transplants." https://www.ispot.tv/ad/dlH3/upmc-living-donor-liver-transplants.

Jarl, Johan, Peter Desatnik, Ulrika Peetz Hansson, Karl Göran Prütz, and Ulf-G Gerdtham. 2018. "Do Kidney Transplantations Save Money? A Study Using a Before-After Design and Multiple Register-Based Data from Sweden." *Clinical Kidney Journal* 11 (2): 283–88. https://doi.org/10.1093/ckj/sfx088.

Katz, Jay. 1993. "Human Experimentation and Human Rights." *Saint Louis University Law Journal* 38:7–33.

"Kidney Failure: A Quirk in the Law Means That America's Kidney Shortage Costs Taxpayers." 2020. *Economist,* February 20, 2020. https://www.economist.com/united-states/2020/02/20/a-quirk-in-the-law-means-that-americas-kidney-shortage-costs-taxpayers.

"Kidney Transplant." n.d. Mayo Clinic. Accessed March 17, 2020. https://www.mayoclinic.org/tests-procedures/kidney-transplant/about/pac-20384777.

"The Kidney Transplant Waiting List." n.d. Living Kidney Donors Network. Accessed March 26, 2020. http://www.lkdn.org/kidney_tx_waiting_list.html.

Klarenbach, Scott, Lianne Barnieh, and John Gill. 2009. "Is Living Kidney Donation the Answer to the Economic Problem of End-Stage Renal Disease?" *Seminars in Nephrology* 29 (5): 533–38. https://doi.org/10.1016/j.semnephrol.2009.06.010.

Koplin, Julian. 2014. "Assessing the Likely Harms to Kidney Vendors in Regulated Organ Markets." *American Journal of Bioethics* 14 (10): 7–18. https://doi.org/10.1080/15265161.2014.947041.

Kritz, Fran. 2017. "Grandfather's Idea for Delayed Kidney Swap Catches On." AARP. October 3, 2017. https://www.aarp.org/health/conditions-treatments/info-2017/grandfather-kidney-donation-program-fd.html.

Kumar, Komal, Elizabeth A. King, Abimereki D. Muzaale, Jonathan M. Konel, Kristina A. Bramstedt, Allan B. Massie, Dorry L. Segev, and Andrew MacGregor Cameron. 2016. "A Smartphone App for Increasing Live Organ Donation." *American Journal of Transplantation* 16 (12): 3548–53. https://doi.org/10.1111/ajt.13961.

Kurland, Rachel. 2017. "Matchmaker, Matchmaker Made a Match for Kidney Transplant." *Jewish Exponent*, July 5, 2017. http://jewishexponent.com/2017/07/05/matchmaker-matchmaker-made-match-kidney-transplant/.

Lentine, Krista L., Ngan N. Lam, and Dorry L. Segev. 2019. "Risks of Living Kidney Donation: Current State of Knowledge on Outcomes Important to Donors." *Clinical Journal of American Society of Nephrology* 14 (4): 597–608. https://doi.org/10.2215/CJN.11220918.

Lentine, Krista L., and Didier Mandelbrot. 2018. "Addressing Disparities in Living Donor Kidney Transplantation." *Clinical Journal of American Society of Nephrology* 13 (12): 1909–11. https://doi.org/10.2215/CJN.06250518.

Lentine, Krista L., and Anita Patel. 2012. "Risks and Outcomes of Living Donation." *Advances in Chronic Kidney Disease* 19 (4): 220–28. https://doi.org/10.1053/j.ackd.2011.09.005.

Lentine, Krista L., Mark A. Schnitzler, Huiling Xiao, Georges Saab, Paolo R. Salvalaggio, David Axelrod, Connie L. Davis, Kevin C. Abbott, and Daniel C. Brennan. 2010. "Racial Variation in Medical Outcomes among Living Kidney Donors." *New England Journal of Medicine* 363:724–32. https://doi.org/10.1056/NEJMoa1000950.

"Living Donors." n.d. National Kidney Registry. Accessed March 17, 2020. https://www.kidneyregistry.org/living_donors.php#overview.

"Living-Donor Transplant." n.d. Mayo Clinic. Accessed March 17, 2020. https://www.mayoclinic.org/tests-procedures/living-donor-transplant/about/pac-20384787.

Marshall, C. Kevin. 2007. "Legality of Alternative Organ Donation Practices under 42 U.S.C. § 274e." US Department of Justice, Office of Legal Counsel, Department of Health and Human Services. March 28, 2007. https://www.justice.gov/sites/default/files/olc/opinions/2007/03/31/organtransplant.pdf.

Martin, Dominque, and Sarah White. 2014. "Risk, Regulation and Financial Incentives for Living Kidney Donors." *American Journal of Bioethics* 14 (10): 46–48. https://doi.org/10.1080/15265161.2014.947045.

Martin, Dominque E., and Gabriel M. Danovitch. 2017. "Banking on Living Kidney Donors—a New Way to Facilitate Donation without Compromising on Ethical Values." *Journal of Medicine & Philosophy* 42 (5): 537–58. https://doi.org/10.1093/jmp/jhx015.

Matthews, Dylan. 2018. "One Simple Change the Government Could Make to Encourage Kidney Donation." *Vox*. December 22, 2018. https://www.vox.com/future-perfect/2018/12/22/18151377/kidney-transplant-waiting-list-national-kidney-foundation.

Medaris Miller, Anna. n.d. "Please Give Me Your Kidney: How to Crowdsource for an Organ." American Transplant Foundation. Accessed March 17, 2020. https://www.americantransplantfoundation.org/2016/07/11/please-give-kidney-crowdsource-organ/.

Merion, Robert M., Valarie B. Ashby, Robert A. Wolfe, Dale A. Distant, Tempie E. Hulbert-Shearon, Robert A. Metzger, Akinlolu O. Ojo, and Friedrich K. Port. 2005. "Deceased-Donor Characteristics and the Survival Benefit of Kidney Transplantation." *Journal of the American Medical Association* 294 (21): 2726–33. https://doi.org/10.1001/jama.294.21.2726.

Meszaros, Liz. 2018. "On This Day in Medical History: First Kidney Transplant Performed by Richard Lawler, MD." MDLinx. https://www.mdlinx.com/internal-medicine/article/1738.

Miller, Jordan, Sinéad Currie, and Ronan E. O'Carroll. 2019. " 'If I Donate My Organs It's a Gift, if You Take Them It's Theft': A Qualitative Study of Planned Donor Decisions Under Opt-Out Legislation." *BMC Public Health* 19 (1): 1463–78. https://doi.org/10.1186/s12889-019-7774-1.

"Mission." n.d. National Living Donor Assistance Center. Accessed March 17, 2020. https://www.livingdonorassistance.org/About-Us/Mission-Background.

"More Transplants Than Ever." 2020. United Network for Organ Sharing. Accessed September 1, 2020. https://unos.org/datatransplant-trends/.

Myers, Beverly, and Wolfgang F. Kuhn. 1988. "Informed Consent Issues in the Cardiac Transplantation Evaluation." *Bulletin of the American Academy of Psychiatry and the Law* 16:59–66.

Naqvi, Syed Ali Anwar, Syed Adibul Hasan Rizvi, Mirza Naqi Zafar, Ejaz Ahmed, B. Ali, K. Mehmood, M. J. Awan, B. Mubarak, and Farida Mazhar. 2008. "Health Status and Renal Function Evaluation of Kidney Vendors: A Report from Pakistan." *American Journal of Transplantation* 8 (7): 1444–50. https://doi.org/10.1111/j.1600-6143.2008.02265.x.

National Living Donor Assistance Center (website). n.d. Accessed March 17, 2020. https://www.livingdonorassistance.org.

National Organ Transplant Act. 1984. Pub. L. No. 98-507 (1984).

Nelson, James Lindemann. 2005. "Trust and Transplants." *American Journal of Bioethics* 5 (4): 26–28. https://doi.org/10.1080/15265160500194261.

O'Keefe, Linda M., Anna Ramond, Clare Oliver-Williams, Petere Willeit, Ellie Paige, Patrick Trotter, Johnathan Evans, et al. 2018. "Mid- and Long-Term Health Risks in Living Kidney Donors: A Systematic Review and Meta-Analysis." *Annals of Internal Medicine* 168 (4): 276–84. https://doi.org/10.7326/M17-1235.

"Organ Donation Again Sets Record in 2019." 2020. News. United Network for Organ Sharing. January 9, 2020. https://unos.org/news/organ-donation-sets-record-in-2019/.

"Organ, Eye and Tissue Donation Statistics." n.d. Donate Life America. Accessed March 17, 2020. https://www.donatelife.net/statistics/.

"Organs." n.d. Transplant Living. United Network for Organ Sharing. Accessed March 17, 2020. https://transplantliving.org/living-donation/organs/.

Parker, Ian. 2004. "The Gift: Zell Kravinsky Gave Away Millions. But Somehow It Wasn't Enough." *New Yorker*, July 26, 2004, 54–63. https://www.newyorker.com/magazine/2004/08/02/the-gift-ian-parker.

Picoult, Jodi. 2004. *My Sister's Keeper.* New York: Atria Books.

"Polycystic Kidney Disease." n.d. Genetics Home Reference. US National Library of Medicine, National Institutes of Health. Accessed March 18, 2020. https://ghr.nlm.nih.gov/condition/polycystic-kidney-disease#statistics.

Pope, Adam. 2018. "Nation's Longest Single-Site Kidney Chain Reaches 100." UAB News. University of Alabama at Birmingham. July 30, 2018. https://www.uab.edu/news/health/item/9638-nation-s-longest-single-site-kidney-chain-reaches-100.

Pope, Adam. 2019. "Living Donor Navigators Are Crucial Part of Organ Transplant." UAB News. University of Alabama at Birmingham. April 29, 2019. https://www.uab.edu/news/people/item/10442-living-donor-navigators-are-crucial-part-of-organ-transplant.

"Risks of Surgery." n.d. National Kidney Foundation. Accessed March 17, 2020. https://www.kidney.org/transplantation/livingdonors/risks-of-surgery.

Ross, Lainie F., David T. Rubin, Mark Siegler, Michelle A. Josephson, J. Richard Thistlethwaite, and E. Steve Woodle. 1997. "Ethics of a Paired Kidney Exchange Program." *New England Journal of Medicine* 336:1752–54. https://doi.org/10.1056/NEJM199706123362412.

Saunders, Ben. 2012. "Opt-Out Organ Donation without Presumptions." *Journal of Medical Ethics* 38:69–72. https://doi.org/10.1136/medethics-2011-100039.

Seelig, Beth J., and Lisa S. Rosof. 2001. "Normal and Pathological Altruism." *Journal of the American Psychoanalytic Association* 49 (3): 933–59. https://doi.org/10.1177/00030651010490031901.

Shapiro, Benson P., V. Kasturi Rangan, and John Sviokla. 2004. "Staple Yourself to an Order." 2004. *Harvard Business Review*, July–August 2004. https://hbr.org/2004/07/staple-yourself-to-an-order.

Singal, Deepa, Mitchell Mickey, and Patricia Terasaki. 1969. "Serotyping for Homotransplantation. 23. Analysis of Kidney Transplants from Parental versus Sibling Donors." *Transplantation* 7 (4): 246–58.

Spital, Aaron. 1989. "Unconventional Living Kidney Donors—Attitudes and Use among Transplant Centers." *Transplantation* 48:243–48. https://doi.org/10.1097/00007890-198908000-00012.

Spital, Aaron. 1994. "Unrelated Living Kidney Donors." *Transplantation* 57 (12): 1722–26. https://journals.lww.com/transplantjournal/Abstract/1994/06270/UNRELATED_LIVING_KIDNEY_DONORS__An_Update_of.6.aspx.

Spital, Aaron. 2000. "Evolution of Attitudes at U.S. Transplant Centers toward Kidney Donation by Friends and Altruistic Strangers." *Transplantation* 69 (8): 1728–31. https://doi.org/10.1097/00007890-200004270-00035.

Spital, Aaron, and David Z. Levine. 1998. "When a Stranger Offers a Kidney: Ethical Issues in Living Organ Donation." *American Journal of Kidney Disease* 32 (4): 676–91. https://doi.org/10.1016/s0272-6386(98)70037-x.

"Statistics." n.d. The Kidney Project. University of California San Francisco. Accessed June 21, 2019. https://pharm.ucsf.edu/kidney/need/statistics.

Starzl, Thomas E., Lawrence Brettschneider, Alfred J. Martin, Jr., Carl G. Groth, Herve Blanchard, George V. Smith, and Israel Penn. 1968. "Organ Transplantation, Past and Present." *Surgical Clinics of North America* 48 (4): 817–38. https://doi.org/10.1016/s0039-6109(16)38585-1.

Starzl, Thomas E., Shunzaburo Iwatsuki, Byers W. Shaw Jr., Robert D. Gordon, and Carlos O. Esquivel. 1985. "Immunosuppression and Other Nonsurgical Factors in the Improved Results of Liver Transplantation." *Seminars in Liver Disease* 5 (4): 334–43. https://doi.org/10.1055/s-2008-1040630.

Steinberg, David. 2003. "Kidneys and the Kindness of Strangers." *Health Affairs* 22:184–89. https://doi.org/10.1377/hlthaff.22.4.184.

Steinbrook, Robert. 2005. "Public Solicitation of Organ Donors." *New England Journal of Medicine* 353:441–44. https://doi.org/10.1056/NEJMp058151.

"Ten Years Since First Non-Directed Donation in the UK." 2017. Give a Kidney. http://www.giveakidney.org/2017/latest-news/10-years-since-the-first-non-directed-donation-in-the-uk/.

Thorwald, Jürgen. 1971. *The Patients.* New York: Harcourt Brace Jovanovich.

Torres, Ana-Marie, Finesse Wong, Sophie Pearson, Sandy Weinberg, John P. Roberts, Nancy L. Ascher, Chris E. Freise, and Brian K. Lee. 2019. "Bi-Organ Paired Exchange—Sentinel Case of a Liver-Kidney Swap." *American Journal of Transplantation* 19 (9): 2646–49. https://doi.org/10.1111/ajt.15386.

"Transplants by Donor Type." n.d. National Data. Organ Procurement and Transplantation Network. US Department of Health and Human Services. Accessed February 21, 2020. https://optn.transplant.hrsa.gov/data/view-data-reports/national-data/.

"Transplants by Donor Type, Center." n.d. National Data. Organ Procurement and Transplantation Network. US Department of Health and Human Services. Accessed January 7, 2020. https://optn.transplant.hrsa.gov/data/view-data-reports/national-data/.

"Transplant Trends." n.d. United Network for Organ Sharing. Accessed March 17, 2020. https://unos.org/data/transplant-trends/.

Truog, Robert D. 2005. "The Ethics of Organ Donation by Living Donors." *New England Journal of Medicine* 353:444–46. https://doi.org/10.1056/NEJMp058155.

Truog, Robert D., and Walter M. Robinson. 2003. "Role of Brain Death and the Dead-Donor Rule in the Ethics of Organ Transplantation." *Critical Care Medicine* 31 (9): 2391–96. https://doi.org/10.1097/01.CCM.0000090869.19410.3C.

UnitedHealth Group. 2016. "UnitedHealthcare Will Reimburse Kidney Donors' Travel Expenses, Expanding Life-Saving Access to Kidney Transplants." Press release. June 13, 2016. https://www.unitedhealthgroup.com/newsroom/2016/0613kidneydonortravelexpenses.html.

Wang, Jeffrey H., Melissa A. Skeans, and Ajay K. Israni. 2016. "Current Status of Kidney Transplant Outcomes: Dying to Survive." *Advances in Chronic Kidney Disease* 23 (5): 281–86. https://doi.org/10.1053/j.ackd.2016.07.001.

Index